THE PSYCHIATRIC TREATMENT
OF ALZHEIMER'S DISEASE

Report No. 125

THE PSYCHIATRIC TREATMENT OF ALZHEIMER'S DISEASE

Formulated by the
Committee on Aging

Group for the Advancement of Psychiatry

BRUNNER/MAZEL *Publishers* • New York

Library of Congress Cataloging-in-Publication Data

The Psychiatric treatment of Alzheimer's disease / formulated
  by the Committee on Aging, Group for the Advancement of
  Psychiatry.

     p.   cm. — (Report; no. 125)
     Includes bibliographies and index
     ISBN 0-87630-519-2
     1. Alzheimer's disease—Treatment.   2. Psychotherapy.
I. Group for the Advancement of Psychiatry.   Committee on
Aging.   II. Series : Report (Group for the Advancement of
Psychiatry : 1984); no. 125.
     [DNLM : 1. Alzheimer's Disease — therapy.   W1 RE209BR
no. 125 / WM 220 P974]
RC321.G7 no. 125
[RC523]
616.89 s — dc 19
[618.97'683]
DNLM / DLC
for Library of Congress   88-14618
                                                  CIP

Copyright © 1988 by the Group for the Advancement of Psychiatry

Published by
BRUNNER/MAZEL, INC.
19 Union Square West
New York, New York 10003

MANUFACTURED IN THE UNITED STATES OF AMERICA

10   9   8   7   6   5   4   3   2   1

STATEMENT OF PURPOSE

THE GROUP FOR THE ADVANCEMENT OF PSYCHIATRY has a membership of approximately 300 psychiatrists, most of whom are organized in the form of a number of working committees. These committees direct their efforts toward the study of various aspects of psychiatry and the application of this knowledge to the fields of mental health and human relations.

Collaboration with specialists in other disciplines has been and is one of GAP's working principles. Since the formation of GAP in 1946, its members have worked closely with such other specialists as anthropologists, biologists, economists, statisticians, educators, lawyers, nurses, psychologists, sociologists, social workers, and experts in mass communication, philosophy, and semantics. GAP envisages a continuing program of work according to the following aims:

1. To collect and appraise significant data in the fields of psychiatry, mental health, and human relations;
2. To reevaluate old concepts and to develop and test new ones;
3. To apply the knowledge thus obtained for the promotion of mental health and good human relations.

GAP is an independent group, and its reports represent the composite findings and opinions of its members only, guided by its many consultants.

The Psychiatric Treatment of Alzheimer's Disease was formulated by the Committee on Public Education. The members of this committee are listed on page vii. The members of the other GAP committees, as well as additional membership categories and current and past officers of GAP, are listed on pp. 000–000.

Committee on Aging
Group for the Advancement of Psychiatry

Gene D. Cohen, *Chairman*

Eric D. Caine
Charles M. Gaitz
Gabe J. Maletta
Robert J. Nathan
George H. Pollock
Kenneth M. Sakauye
Charles A. Shamoian
F. Conyers Thompson, Jr.

Joanne Ahola, *Fellow*
Catharine S. C. Buttinger, *Fellow*
Andrew F. Leuchter, *Fellow*

CONTENTS

THE PSYCHIATRIC TREATMENT
OF ALZHEIMER'S DISEASE

OVERVIEW

Alzheimer's disease continues to be poorly understood clinically—from two critically important and intersecting vantage points:

1. Although there is no cure for Alzheimer's disease, *there is treatment.* The patient's symptoms and suffering can be alleviated, and coping skills and dignity in living through the course of the disorder can be enhanced. At the same time, clinical interventions can help to mitigate the very high degree of family stress and reactive depression that can accompany Alzheimer's disease, thereby improving the quality of life for the family as a whole.
2. The major clinical problems that characterize the natural history of Alzheimer's disease are mostly *behavioral and psychosocial* in nature, well into its clinical course. Indeed, the National Institutes of Health Consensus Development Conference statement, "Differential Diagnosis Of Dementing Diseases," pointed out that "dementia is primarily a behavioral diagnosis" (US Department of Health and Human Services, 1987).

The absence of characteristic somatic symptoms and laboratory findings is what makes the diagnosis of Alzheimer's disease so difficult. But the nature of the behavioral and psychosocial problems defines treatment opportunities. This is where these two vantage points intersect: *Treatments are available to modify the behavioral dysfunctions that are a part of Alzheimer's disease.* The benefits for both the patient and the family can be pronounced.

With Alzheimer's disease, because a major part of the clinical focus is on behavioral dysfunction and psychosocial stress, psychiatric expertise and mental health interventions are of enormous value (Merriam et al., 1988; Terri, Larson & Reifler, 1988). Thus the thrust of this Group for the Advancement of Psychiatry report is on elaborating the psychiatric treatment of Alzheimer's disease.

The introduction presents a synopsis of some of the major points, while briefly reviewing the contributions of basic science in the search for the cause of Alzheimer's disease. Chapters on Clinicopathologic Correlations, Diagnosis, and Treatment follow, with an emphasis on psychiatric skill. To make the issues and opportunities for treatment yet more concrete, ten case examples are presented, with key clinical concepts delineated in each. References are listed with each chapter, while a general Bibliography is included at the end. Finally, the Appendix presents five rating scales for assessing different patient characteristics and levels of functioning.

This report should provide the reader with a considerably better understanding of opportunities for and approaches to clinical intervention in Alzheimer's disease, and a better awareness of the important contributions that psychiatric skills can make. Health care providers in general can benefit from this knowledge, both in their own interventions and in seeking consultative assistance.

REFERENCES

Merriam, A.E., Aronson, M.K., Gaston, P., Wey, S., & Katz, I. (1988). The psychiatric symptoms of Alzheimer's disease. *JAGS, 36,* 1–6.

Terri, L., Larson, E., & Reifler, B.V. (1988). Behavioral disturbance in dementia of the Alzheimer's type. *JAGS, 36,* 7–12.

US Department of Health and Human Services. (1987). Differential diagnosis of dementing diseases. *National Institutes of Health Consensus Development Conference Statement, 6*(11), 1–27.

1
INTRODUCTION

HISTORY

In 1906, a psychiatrist by the name of Alois Alzheimer presented what would become a classic case and paper to the Association of Southwest German Specialists in Mental Diseases. The next year he published the paper on what would soon after be called "Alzheimer's disease." An excerpt follows from the patient's history obtained during her psychiatric hospitalization.

> A woman 51 years of age exhibited ideas of jealousy against her husband as the first notable symptom. Soon a rapidly progressing loss of memory became apparent; she could no longer find her way around her home, dragged objects back and forth, hid them; at times she believed someone wanted to kill her and began to shout loudly. (Alzheimer, 1907)

From a psychiatric viewpoint Alzheimer's disease (AD) is of enormous interest because, while it is a devastating brain disorder with major neuroanatomical and neurochemical alterations, most of the major clinical problems and symptoms that result are behavioral (generically speaking) in nature, well into its clinical course (Cohen, 1987). This unusual aspect of the disorder largely explains the difficulty in making its diagnosis and why misdiagnosis is so common; many other disorders, ranging from depression to drug side effects, can produce similar behavioral manifestations. This also sets Alzheimer's disease apart from many other brain diseases. With a stroke, observable physical signs—nerve, motor, or muscular changes—are typically observed. Not so with AD, where the clinical manifestations are cognitive, behavioral, and psychological, with an absence of specific findings on physical examinations and laboratory tests.

More specifically, clinical issues of high psychiatric relevance in AD fall into four general areas: 1) cognitive dysfunction; 2) problem behaviors; 3) psychological symptoms; and 4) psychosocial stress. Cognitive dysfunction in AD is most apparent in impairment of memory and intellect. Problem behaviors include agitation and wandering, the latter often raising the question of nursing home placement. Psychological symptoms include depression and delusions. Psychosocial difficulties are reflected in the great stress experienced by families, with clinical depression disturbingly common in the caregiving relatives of AD patients. Suicide is most frequent in the elderly in general, so its risk should be monitored closely in both the Alzheimer patient and the spouse—both of whom come under considerable stress at different points along the course of the disorder. It is these problems that determine the clinical need and opportunity for psychiatric interventions and treatment planning.

The classification of Alzheimer's disease in DSM-III-R (APA, 1987) represents an attempt to define subtypes so as to structure the way one views symptoms for treatment purposes. DSM-III-R classifies the disorder as follows:

Primary degenerative dementia of the Alzheimer type, senile onset

> 290.30 with delirium
> 290.20 with delusions
> 290.21 with depression
> 290.00 uncomplicated

The cognitive, behavioral, psychological, and psychosocial aspects of AD are all illustrated in Alzheimer's original case. Cognition was impaired, as reflected in the description of the patient's "rapidly progressing loss of memory." Her general behavior revealed difficulty with coping skills ("she could no longer find her way around her home") and maladaptive responses (she "dragged objects back and forth, hid them"). Psychologically, she manifested paranoid delusions in her psychotic concerns that "someone wanted to kill her." The psychosocial stress that can emerge in interpersonal relationships and family interactions was portrayed in how she "exhibited ideas of jealousy against her husband."

The disorder was named "Alzheimer's disease" by Emil Kraepelin, one of the leading figures in the history of psychiatry. At the time, Alois Alzheimer was Head of the Psychiatric Research Laboratory at the Institute of which Kraepelin was Director. Alzheimer finished his career as Chairman of the Department of Psychiatry at the University of Breslau (Schiller, 1970; Talbott, 1970). Alzheimer and others then viewed the condition as limited to middle-aged patients. Another description, "presenile dementia," was used to distinguish these patients from older patients with what had been called "senile dementia." When the same neuropathological picture was later identified in patients over as well as under 65 years old, the term "Alzheimer's disease" became used for both age groups.

DEFINITION

Alzheimer's disease (AD) is a brain disorder of unknown cause, characterized by an insidious onset and a progressive, irreversible loss of intellectual function. Terminology varies in references to this disorder. DSM-III-R refers to the disease as "primary degenerative dementia (PDD) of the Alzheimer type." Its clinical diagnosis is one of both exclusion and the passage of time to demonstrate deterioration. All other specific causes of dementia must be ruled out by the clinical history, physical examination, laboratory tests, psychometric and other special studies *and* continued decline must be demonstrated over time (McKhann et al., 1984).

Characteristic neuropathological findings have been classically described (Katzman, 1986). These include the microscopic brain tissue formations of senile plaques (neuritic plaques), neurofibrillary tangles, and granulovacuolar degeneration of neurons in the cerebral cortex. The brains of AD patients below and over age 65 reveal these findings on autopsy examinations. Computer-assisted tomography (CT Scan) changes become more evident as the disease progresses—not necessarily apparent early on. Over time, the CT Scan may reveal an atrophied brain with widened cortical sulci and enlarged cerebral ventricles. Other pathological findings, including nerve cell degeneration in the nucleus basalis of Meynert within the subcortical area of the brain (Whitehouse et al., 1981) and reduced levels of cerebral RNA (Sajdel-Sulkowska & Marotta, 1984), have been described, but from a practical clinical standpoint, the classical changes typically suffice for a tissue diagnosis. A specific diagnostic marker on clinical examination of Alzheimer patients in general, however, has yet to be found, although intensive investigations are currently underway to identify such a marker. There have been preliminary reports of a protein (A-68) being in considerably greater quantities in Alzheimer brains than in normals and being isolated in cerebrospinal fluid, attracting considerable interest as the basis of a possible specific clinical test to diagnose the disorder (Wolozin et al., 1986). The discovery of a genetic marker on chromosome 21 in selected families with AD may also lead to a diagnostic marker, at least in those families with an autosomal dominant form of the disorder (St. George-Hyslop et al., 1987).

The average course of the disease from onset to death is about 5–10 years, with a range from under 2 to over 20 years. Hence, the specific problems, along with the rate and severity of decline, vary with the individual. Because AD may so radically alter longevity, many have regarded the disorder as the fourth or fifth leading cause of death (Katzman, Terry & Bick, 1978).

It is estimated that between 2% and 6% of people over the age of 65 have AD; a considerably smaller percentage have an onset prior to 65 years of age (Reisberg, 1983). The incidence and prevalence increases with advancing age, especially after the late 70s. It is estimated that at least half the people in nursing homes in the United States have Alzheimer's disease or a related disorder, with costs in excess of 13 billion dollars incurred annually for this group alone.

For reasons that are not clear, AD may be more common in

women than in men; this difference may not be explained entirely by the increased longevity of older women resulting in many more women than men at advanced ages (women outnumber men 2:1 by age 85). A familial pattern has been described by various investigators, suggesting that heredity may be of some importance; other researchers emphasize how rudimentary our understanding is of genetic aspects of the disorder (Davies, 1986). While the discovery of a genetic marker on chromosome 21 does establish a genetic basis with *some* families, available data indicate that the overall likelihood of a first degree relative of an Alzheimer patient developing AD may only be four times greater than that in the general population, where the risk is well below 1%. Of course, many disorders have a genetic potential that is either never expressed, partially expressed, or only expressed in combination with other risk factors. There have also been a few reports of a possible association between serious head injuries and the later onset of Alzheimer's disease (Mortimer et al., 1985). To date no other risk factors have been unequivocally identified for AD.

NORMAL COGNITIVE CHANGES WITH AGING

Not all memory changes in later life are pathognomonic of dementia or mental disorder. Many memory changes are only temporary, such as those that occur with bereavement or any stressful situation that makes it difficult to concentrate. In fact, older people are often accused or accuse themselves of memory changes that are not really taking place. If a person in his thirties misplaces keys or a wallet, forgets the name of a neighbor, or calls one sibling by another's name, nobody gives it a second thought. But the same normal forgetfulness for people in their seventies may raise unjustifiable concern. A brief review of the literature on normal cognitive function with aging is revealing.

Normative Aging Studies on Cognition

Owens (1966) reported on a longitudinal study of intellectual performance in 96 men, average age 61, who had initially been tested in 1919 as freshman at Iowa State University. The key finding of this study was that, on the average, little change occurred in intellectual test scores as these men aged from 50 to 60 years. An earlier report by Owens (1953) had shown increments in verbal ability and total score of intellectual performance as these men moved from age 20 to 50, though numerical ability showed a slight decline. These longitudinal studies were among the first to raise serious doubts about presumed normal decline in mental abilities with advancing age, which had been inferred from earlier cross-sectional studies.

A 12-year longitudinal study of men, median age 71, was initiated in 1955 at the National Institute of Mental Health (Granick & Patterson, 1971). The aim of the study was to examine a wide range of variables in individuals of advanced age in whom disease was absent or minimal, in an attempt to differentiate the impact of aging from that of illness on older adults. Of note in these healthy aging subjects, as they moved on the average from their 70s to their 80s, was that while various intellectual functions declined, others improved. Speed in carrying out different operations declined; quality of sentence completions declined. On the other hand, vocabulary and picture arrangement both improved. In terms of everyday living, these findings suggest that certain activities requiring quick reactions or a high degree of precision might not be carried out as well by older adults in general, but the ability to understand one's situation and to learn from new experiences is maintained in later life. Moreover, the study found that decrements in intellectual performance with advancing age were significantly greater in subjects who also developed arteriosclerotic cardiovascular disease than in subjects who remained healthy. This study illustrates the impact of illness on intellectual functioning with aging, but shows that intellectual functioning is maintained in older healthy individuals.

Many *"normal"* older individuals experience memory difficulties that have been described as "age-associated memory impairment" (Crook et al., 1986) or "benign senescent forgetfulness" (Kral, 1978).

How personally disturbing these symptoms are varies greatly with different individuals, some of whom may need and benefit from psychotherapy. At the same time, *serious* memory difficulties should not be dismissed as a concomitant of normal aging. Since rigorous studies on intelligence in later life show that healthy people who stay intellectually active maintain a sharp mind throughout the life cycle, noticeable decline should be explored for an underlying problem (Birren & Sloane, 1980). In the presence of such decline, the diagnosis of Alzheimer's disease must be considered. While the diagnosis of AD can be very difficult, particularly early in its clinical course, its etiology has remained completely elusive.

THE SEARCH FOR CAUSE

Alzheimer's disease has emerged as one of the great mysteries in modern day medicine, with many clues but no answers as to its cause. The quest to uncover its etiology has the air of a veritable whodunit. There have been at least six prominent theories as to the genesis of Alzheimer's disease (Katzman, 1983): 1) vascular; 2) slow virus; 3) autoimmune; 4) chemical; 5) genetic; and 6) normal aging.

Vascular Theory

Hardening of the arteries, or cerebroarteriosclerosis, contrary to considerable popular belief, is not the cause of Alzheimer's disease. Arteriosclerosis is more associated with multi-infarct dementia or stroke. The hyperbaric oxygen chamber is a treatment technique whose use was based upon an arteriosclerotic hypothesis, and accordingly has proved unsuccessful. A major clinical lesson from this research is how important it is for the practitioner to be as much aware of which interventions do not work as which do work in treatment approaches for Alzheimer's disease. The ramifications for patient and family alike are clearly profound.

Slow Virus, or Unconventional Transmissible Agent Theory

While a slow acting viral cause has been identified for some brain disorders that closely resemble Alzheimer's disease (e.g., Creutzfeld-Jakob disease), and while there are histological findings in AD brains that some investigators hypothesize represent changes caused by a virus, a slow virus has not been unequivocally isolated from those with AD (Gibbs & Gajdusek, 1978).

Autoimmune Theory

Though antibrain antibodies have been identified in the brains of those with AD, their significance is not understood (Nandy, 1978).

Chemical Theories

Chemical Deficiencies (e.g., acetylcholine and other neurotransmitters). Findings of diminished levels of the neurotransmitter acetylcholine in brains of patients with Alzheimer's disease and the clinical manifestation of altered intellectual functioning due to anticholinergic effects of certain drugs on the CNS have led to a number of pharmacologic trials with agents that enhance cholinergic activity. Such drugs have varied from precursors (e.g., lecithin) involved in the synthesis of acetylcholine to enzyme inhibitors (e.g., physostigmine and THA) that interfere with the metabolic breakdown of the neurotransmitter (Reisberg, 1983). Drug trials have been initiated in attempts to elevate the levels of other neurotransmitters (e.g., norepinephrine, serotonin, dopamine, somatostatin) also found to be diminished in AD (Goodnick, Gershon & Salzman, 1984). Results to date have been of interest to investigators who see small but statistically significant results as suggesting that research is moving in the right direction; however, results have not as yet been sufficiently significant clinically (Funkenstein et al., 1981). Enthusiastic reports on drug trials with memory-enhancing agents for Alzheimer patients represent the excitement of the research community, which feels it may be on the right *trail,* not excitement among clinicians, who have not yet seen clinical improvement with these drugs.

Chemical Excesses (e.g., toxic accumulations of aluminum). Although various studies have shown increased levels of aluminum in the brains of Alzheimer's disease victims, others have not (Terry, 1985). While some investigators have hypothesized that aluminum may have a part in the genesis of AD, most have regarded aluminum as an *effect* of the disorder rather than its *cause*. Instead of inducing neuropathological changes, aluminum more likely accumulates in response to such changes. Among the findings that do not implicate aluminum in AD are those showing that neuropathological changes induced by aluminum differ from those observed in Alzheimer's disease. Others regard the build-up of aluminum as an epiphenomenon and point to AD patient samples where brain aluminum levels are not elevated.

Genetic Theory

As already alluded to, genetic aspects of this disorder are confusing. A disorder can be familial and not genetic, congenital (e.g., from prenatal factors) and not hereditary, or hereditary and not clinically expressed. Moreover, there may be certain forms of a disorder that are hereditary, and others not. Genetic interest in AD has been further stirred, however, by an association between the occurrence of Alzheimer's disease and Down's Syndrome among different members of the same family. Although a basic understanding of this finding remains elusive, it has led to efforts to identify a genetic marker for AD on chromosome 21—the chromosome affected in Down's syndrome. Such efforts have gained additional momentum due to the existence of a small group of families where an autosomal dominant trait appears to be operating, suggesting that there may be genetic subtypes of the disorder (Briley, Chopin & Moret, 1986). Genetic subtypes now appear even more likely with the discovery of a genetic linkage marker on chromosome 21 in the autosomal dominant families. But the extent of genetic and hereditary involvement in families as a whole with AD remains unclear because of the vast number affected with this disorder who do not manifest autosomal dominant disease patterns or clear-cut genetic features (Davies, 1986).

Normal Aging—The Largely Dismissed Theory

In the past, when Alzheimer's disease was referred to as senility, it was regarded as part of normal aging, or an accelerated variant thereof. Investigators point out, however, that if AD were simply accelerated aging, then numerous other changes characteristic of the aging process should also be exaggerated in addition to the mental impairment. But this is one of the multiple tragedies of AD, that one can have marked cognitive deterioration juxtaposed with excellent physical health. The findings of a genetic defect on chromosome 21 in a specific group of families also speak against AD being a variant of normal aging.

TREATMENT

Two critical crossroads reached in the approach to treatment for Alzheimer's disease are: 1) recognition of AD as a disorder demanding treatment as opposed to an inevitable concomitant of normal aging; and 2) realization that in developing interventions for a major illness or disability, the concept of care can be as important as that of cure (Miller & Cohen, 1981). Moreover, the clinical course of Alzheimer's disease is commonly marked by various symptoms that can compound the memory impairment of the disorder, making the person worse than would be expected from the dementia alone. Depression and delusions can affect the AD patient in this way, causing what has been referred to as *"excess disability"* states—clinical conditions that can be alleviated with proper treatment. Indeed, this highlights one of the truly extraordinary phenomena that can be observed in Alzheimer's disease. Through the alleviation of an excess disability state in AD, actual clinical improvement can result for a period of time in the course of the disorder, in the face of an underlying progressive pathological process (Cohen, 1984). This phenomenon is discussed in more detail in the chapter on treatment and is illustrated in a number of the case examples to follow.

In general, the behavioral problems in Alzheimer's disease play a major role in influencing how well and how long a person with AD can remain in the community and out of a nursing home. To the extent that a treatment plan is developed based on a problem-oriented approach focused on these behavioral issues, patient suffering can be diminished and functional capacities maximized at different stages of the illness. Meanwhile, family burden is reduced and the quality of life enhanced for all involved. The patient is helped in this way to live through the illness with greater dignity and less discomfort. All of this is treatment, in the traditional sense.

The financing of treatment for AD has, until recently, represented a serious problem. It was in part in recognition of the role and potential impact of psychiatric intervention in Alzheimer's disease that "the most important change in Medicare coverage for mental disorders since the inception of Medicare" more than 20 years ago was announced in the fall of 1984 (Goldman, Cohen & Davis, 1985). In September of that year, a major Task Force Report on Alzheimer's Disease was released by the US Department of Health and Human Services.Within the report there was a special financing recommendation that was announced as being implemented in conjunction with the release of the report. The purpose of the recommendation was to remove limitations on services (for Alzheimer's disease and related disorders) provided outside the hospital setting. Specifically, the recommendation, which is now supposed to be in force, reads as follows:

> Current Medicare statute limits medically appropriate physician services provided outside of the hospital setting for patients with Alzheimer's disease when coded as a mental disorder. The Department should clarify that, except for psychotherapy, physician treatment services for patients with Alzheimer's disease and related disorders are not subject to the $250 limitations. In other words, in determining whether services for these patients are subject to the limit, the nature of the physician's service is the deciding factor, not the diagnostic code. Therefore, physician treatment services provided outside the hospital setting for patients with Alzheimer's disease

and related disorders coded 290.X (in DSM-III and ICD-9) should be reimbursed in the same manner as services for Alzheimer's disease coded 331 (ICD-9). (US Department of Health and Human Services, 1984, p. xv)

The intent of this administrative change was to correct an inconsistency where reimbursement for the same service differed depending on which diagnostic code for the treatment of Alzheimer's disease was used (290.X vs. 331), although both codes refer to Alzheimer's disease and related disorders. The intent, too, was to reimburse for office visits for the medical management of Alzheimer's disease (including pharmacotherapy and other nonpsychotherapy psychiatric treatment interventions) on an 80:20 reimbursement/copayment formula, as opposed to the $250.00 limit and 50:50 reimbursement/copayment formula that has applied to the treatment of mental disorders under Medicare. Psychotherapy for Alzheimer's disease is still reimbursable, though under the 50:50 reimbursement/copayment restrictions. Medicare changes during 1988 and 1989, however, increase the cap on the federal share for psychotherapy coverage from $250.00 to $1,100.00 a year. These overall changes should significantly improve the ability of patients suffering from Alzheimer's disease or a related disorder to seek state-of-the-art clinical intervention.

PRESENT DEVELOPMENTS

While Alzheimer's disease remains a mystery, with its cause and cure not yet found, there is considerable excitement and hope about truly new frontier research presently unfolding before us in numerous settings (Bartus, 1986; Davies & Wolozin, 1987; Reifler & Larson, 1988; Wurtman, 1985). The pieces to the puzzle of Alzheimer's disease continue to increase and to connect. Still, for the major part of the 20th century, the challenge of and curiosity about Alzheimer's disease has focused almost exclusively on unraveling the significance of the plaques and tangles described in Alzheimer's (1907) paper and on other neuropathological findings viewed as potential leads in the pursuit of etiology. Finally, some four score years later, the behavioral problems originally described by Alzheimer, which lead to excess disability and form much of the basis for treatment in Alzheimer's disease, are becoming better understood. The potential role for psychiatric interventions in addressing these problems is enormous.

REFERENCES

Alzheimer, A. (1907). Ueber eine eigenartige erkrankung der hirnrinde. *Allegemeine Zeitschrift für Psychiatrie Psychisch-Gerichtlich Medizin*, 146–148.

American Psychiatric Association. *Diagnostic and statistical manual of mental disorders* (3rd ed. rev.). Washington, DC: APA.

Bartus, R.T. (Ed.) (1986). Special issue: Controversial topics on Alzheimer's disease: Intersecting crossroads. *Neurobiology of Aging, 7*(6).

Birren, J.E., & Sloane, R.B. (Eds.). (1980). *Handbook of mental health and aging*. Englewood Cliffs, NJ: Prentice-Hall.

Briley, M., Chopin, P., & Moret, C. (1986). New concepts in Alzheimer's disease. *Neurobiology of Aging, 7*(1).

Cohen, G.D. (1987). Alzheimer's disease. In G.L. Maddox (Ed.), *Encyclopedia of Aging* (pp. 27–30). New York: Springer.

Cohen, G.D. (1984). The mental health professional and the Alzheimer patient. *Hospital and Community Psychiatry, 35*(2), 115–116.

Crook, T., Bartus, R.T., Ferris, S.H., Whitehouse, P., Cohen, G.D., & Gershon, S. (1986). Age-associated memory impairment: Proposed diagnostic criteria and measures of clinical change—Report of a National Institute of Mental Health work group. *Developmental Neuropsychology, 2*(4), 261–276.

Davies, P. (1986). The genetics of Alzheimer's disease: A review and a discussion of the implications. *Neurobiology of Aging, 7,* 459–466.

Davies, P., & Wolozin, B.L. (1987). Recent advances in the neurochemistry of Alzheimer's disease. *Journal of Clinical Psychiatry, 48,* 23–30.

Funkenstein, H.H., Hicks, R., Dysken, M.W., & Davis, J.M. (1981). Drug treatment of cognitive impairment in Alzheimer's disease and the late life dementias. In N.E. Miller & G.D. Cohen (Eds.), *Clinical aspects of Alzheimer's disease and senile dementia* (pp. 139–160). New York: Raven Press.

Gibbs, C.J., & Gajdusek, D.C. (1978). Subacute spongiform virus encephalopathies: The transmissible virus dementias. In R. Katzman & R.D. Terry (Eds.), *Alzheimer's disease: Senile dementia and related disorders*. New York: Raven Press.

Goldman, H.H., Cohen, G.D., & Davis, M. (1985). Expanded Medicare outpatient coverage for Alzheimer's disease. *Hospital & Community Psychiatry, 36,* 939–942.

Goodnick, P., Gershon, S., & Salzman, C. (1984). Dementia and memory loss in the elderly. In C. Salzman (Ed.), *Clinical geriatric psycho-pharmacology* (pp. 171–198). New York: McGraw-Hill Book.

Granick, S. & Patterson, R.D. (1971). *Human aging II: An eleven-year follow-up biomedical and behavioral study.* DHEW Publication No. (HSM) 71-9037.

Katzman, R. (Ed.). (1983). *Biological aspects of Alzheimer's disease.* Cold Spring Harbor Laboratory, NY: Banbury Reports.

Katzman, R. (1986). Alzheimer's disease. *New England Journal of Medicine, 314*(13), 964–973.

Katzman, R., Terry, R.D., & Bick, K.L. (Eds.). (1978). *Alzheimer's disease: Senile dementia and related disorders.* New York: Raven Press.

Kral, V.A. (1978). Benign senescent forgetfulness. In R. Katzman, R.D. Terry, & K.L. Bick (Eds.), *Alzheimer's disease: Senile dementia and related disorders.* New York: Raven Press.

McKhann, G., Drachman, D., Folstein, M., Katzman, R., Price, D., & Stadlan, E.M. (1984). Clinical diagnosis of Alzheimer's disease. *Neurology, 34.*

Miller, N.E., & Cohen, G.D. (Eds.). (1981). *Clinical aspects of Alzheimer's disease and senile dementia.* New York: Raven Press.

Mortimer, J.A., French, L.R., Hutton, J.T., & Schuman, L.M. (1985). Head injury as a risk factor for Alzheimer's disease. *Neurology, 35,* 264–267.

Nandy, K. (1978). Brain-reactive antibodies in aging and senile dementia. In R. Katzman, R.D. Terry, K.L. Bick (Eds.), *Alzheimer's disease: Senile dementia and related disorders* (pp. 503–514). New York: Raven Press.

Owens, W.A. (1953). Age and mental abilities: A longitudinal study. *Genetic Psychology Monographs, 48,* 3–54.

Owens, W.A. (1966). Age and mental abilities: A second follow-up. *Journal of Educational Psychology, 57,* 311–325.

Reifler, B.V., & Larson, E.L. (1988). Excess disability in demented elderly outpatients: The rule of the halves. *JAGS, 36,* 82–83.

Reisberg, B. (Ed.). (1983). *Alzheimer's disease.* New York: Free Press.

Sajdel-Sulkowska, E.M., & Marotta, C.A. (1984). Alzheimer's disease brain: Alterations in RNA levels and in ribonuclease inhibitor complex. *Science, 255,* 947–949.

Schiller, F. (Ed.). (1970). *The founders of neurology* (pp. 315–319). Springfield, IL: Charles C Thomas.

St. George-Hyslop, P.H., Tanzi, R.E., Polinsky, J., Haines, J.L., et al. (1987). The genetic defect causing familial Alzheimer's disease maps on chromosome 21. *Science, 235,* 885–890.

Terry, R.R. (1985). Some unanswered questions about the mechanisms and etiology of Alzheimer's disease. *Danish Medical Bulletin, 32* (Supplement 1), 22–24.

Talbott, J. (1970). *A biographical history of medicine.* New York: Grune & Stratton.

U.S. Department of Health and Human Services Task Force on Alzheimer's Disease. (1984). *DHHS Publication No. (ADM) 84-1323.*

Whitehouse, P.J., Price, D.L., Clark, A.W., Coyle, J.T., & Delong, M.R. (1981). Alzheimer's disease: Evidence for selective loss of cholinergic neurons in the nucleus basalis. *Annals of Neurology, 10,* 122–126.

Wolozin, B.L., Pruchnicki, A., Dickson, D.W., & Davies, P. (1986). A neuronal antigen in the brains of Alzheimer patients. *Science, 232,* 648–650.

Wurtman, R.J. (1985). Alzheimer's disease. *Scientific American, 252,*(1), 62–74.

2

CLINICOPATHOLOGIC CORRELATIONS

Alzheimer's dementia, unlike most other dementias, does not have a clear-cut localizing pattern of brain disease. Rather, it is characterized by its insidious onset, slow, progressive course, and clinical symptomatology of cognitive decline. The disorder is often defined either by characteristic diagnostic test findings (Kahn & Miller, 1978; Rosen et al., 1984), or by the characteristic pattern of progression of the disease (Cummings & Benson, 1983; Reisberg, 1983).

In describing the intellectual changes characteristic of Alzheimer's disease, tests have traditionally focused on assessment of cortical dementia. Cortical performance features, however, are also influenced by performance anxiety and motivational factors, and thoughtful consideration must be applied in the interpretation of results. The primary measurable deficits occur in areas of abstraction, orientation, judgment, memory, and in the associative areas serving language (expressive and comprehensive), skilled movements, and sensory interpretations. However, there has been increasing evidence that Alzheimer's dementia shares features of subcortical and axial dementias as well. Apathy, typified by subcortical dementias such as Huntington's disease (McHugh & Folstein, 1975), is often seen early in the course of Alzheimer's disease (Marco & Randels, 1984). There are also similarities to axial dementias, typified by Wernicke-Korsakoff syndrome, which involve the hippocampus, fornix, mammillary bodies, hypothalamus, and medial temporal lobes. In such dementias there seems to be a striking disturbance in recent memory and new learning, without other intellectual impairments. Early degeneration in these areas has been implicated in Alzheimer's dementia, though it may not represent the primary cause of symptomatology (Marco & Randels, 1984). Thus, there are changes suggestive of a global deterioration beyond simple cortical degeneration. In the early stages, specific decrements and the brain areas involved may vary from patient to patient. These variations may represent different subtypes of the disorder; they also represent areas of further research interest.

The major features and course of the illness have been increasingly detailed in recent years (Cummings & Benson, 1983; Reisberg, 1983). As the disease progresses, treatment goals and objectives need to be redefined according to the levels of understanding or involvement that the patient will be able to master at each stage. The sequence in which higher cognitive functions are lost and behavioral and neurological symptoms appear may even serve as additional clues in establishing a diagnosis (Reisberg, 1983).

The most characteristic changes are seen in five clinical domains: 1) concentration, 2) recent memory, 3) past memory, 4) orientation, and 5) social functioning and self-care. Less consistent changes are seen in specific intellectual functions such as language, visuo-spatial orientation, ideopraxis and motor praxis, or mood and behavior. The general patterns of decline in each of these domains seem to be intercorrelated and to define global stages of functioning (Reisberg, 1983).

In the earliest stage of Alzheimer's dementia, deficits are mainly subjective forgetfulness and generally do not interfere with social or occupational functioning. Changes may not be evident to casual observers or strangers but are clearly evident to the individual and significant others, some of whom may experience considerable stress.

There is often no identifiable deficit other than in comparison to past abilities. The primary early sign is forgetting names of persons and things who were well known to the individual, and forgetting where objects have been placed. In this phase, there may be a below average performance on the WAIS (Wechsler, 1944) and vocabulary subtests. These early stages are not clearly distinguishable from the nonprogressive "normal" variant of aging referred to as "age-associated memory impairment" (Crook et al., 1986) or as "benign senescent forgetfulness" (Kral, 1967). The deficits at this stage are often not perceptible by the clinician unless there is a long past history of interaction with the individual, though some individuals may experience some anxiety or depressive symptomatology in response to perceived cognitive changes.

In the stage of early cognitive decline, decreased performance in demanding employment or social situations is noted. Word-finding and name recall problems become evident. Psychometric tests of memory and concentration will be slightly below average. New learning is sometimes compromised, and there are heightened problems with auditory information (modality effect) (Cummings & Benson, 1983). Such early deficits, however, are difficult to distinguish from those due to anxiety. Personality and social behaviors seem to remain remarkably intact during the early phases of the disease, despite the intellectual deterioration. The capacity for superficial social amenities and exchanges often remains unchanged, and the desire and ability to maintain social ties remains unless there is a concomitant depression. Since memory disturbance is almost always the feature that heralds the onset of the disease, the diagnosis of Alzheimer's disease should be questioned if memory loss is not among the earliest features, or if social or behavioral symptoms are more prominent (Wells, 1979). However, one should also be aware that the isolated finding of memory complaints does not necessarily signify Alzheimer's disease.

During the stage of moderate cognitive decline, amnesia, aphasia, apraxia, carelessness, and spatial and temporal disorientation become more apparent. Patients can no longer perform complex tasks accurately. Three or more errors become evident on the Mental Status Questionnaire (MSQ) (Kahn et al., 1960). Apathy and indifference are common and there is often a motoric restlessness with pacing or other stereotypic responses.

The stage of late cognitive decline is characterized by severely deteriorated intellectual functions. There are deficits in virtually all capacities, and motor disabilities become evident (rigidity, flexion posture, and problems with sphincter control). Diurnal rhythm frequently is disturbed with worsening of symptoms at night and lowered states of arousal. Past knowledge becomes sketchy and awareness of recent events and experiences is lost. Patients make 5–10 errors on the MSQ. Functionally, activities of daily living (ADL) such as dressing, toileting, and bathing are impaired.

The idea of staging reflects the classical observation that the onset of the illness is insidious and involves a progressive loss in language skills, memory and attentional difficulties, abulia (absence of will-power or wish-power), impulsivity, affective lability, and impaired spatial-motor performance. By the middle-to-late phases, Alzheimer's patients seem unable to carry out or follow through on decisions, or maintain a new thought or idea long enough to act upon it effectively (Cummings & Benson, 1983). While remissions do not occur, plateau periods of arrested progression can occur. In general, cognitive skills and behavioral competencies deteriorate at different rates in different people and are not clearly predictable. Also, complete syndromes are not present early in the disease.

Because of the variability, the concept of stages has remained of somewhat limited clinical value. The natural course of Alzheimer's disease seems to be dependent upon a number of factors such as the primary brain areas of degeneration, the patient's general health, preventive social services, family tension, and financial status (Cohen et al., 1984; Zarit & Orr, 1983). Continuing medical and psychosocial evaluations are required to provide information to work with the patient and family throughout the course of dementia.

BEHAVIORAL AND AFFECTIVE CHANGE

In Alzheimer's dementia, behavioral and affective changes often result from organic brain deficits. However, such changes are usually quite variable and may strongly reflect the patient's awareness of deficits and/or pathological attempts to cope with the environment or altered self-perception. Often agitation or hopelessness in the Alzheimer patient reflects the family's reactions to the individual, or the family's expectations of regressed behavior or helplessness. Although differentiation between primary (organic) and secondary (reactive or interpersonal) behavioral effects is often extremely difficult, it is very important to make the distinction in order to determine therapeutic approaches.

Personality change in Alzheimer patients is often discussed in terms of affective disturbance (depression, lability), changes in social perceptiveness or social learning (concreteness and a gradual loss of social skills and empathy), self-regulation or control (impulsivity), stimulus-bound behavior, and increased dependency.

The behavior and "personality" of dementia patients is hardly characteristic and is often described in such contradictory terms as "labile affect," passive, hyperactive, hypoactive, impulsive, rigid, aggressive, docile and dependent, hypersexual, and asexual. In addition, many symptoms are nonspecific such as being negativistic, anxious, irritable, having poor judgment, having low frustration tolerance, and having low self-esteem. The diversity may actually reflect differences in adaptational capacities, which are influenced by many interdependent factors. Impaired judgment, inadequate environmental structures, past life experiences (which have determined expectations and psychological defense styles), and the nature of external stressors may be even more important associations to behavioral disturbances than neuroanatomic brain deficits in this disorder. While the delusions, depression, or other psychiatric disturbances seen with the disorder may be part of the disorder per se, they could also represent coexisting, independent psychiatric diagnoses. They can also represent pseudodementia (discussed in the chapter on diagnosis) misdiagnosed as Alzheimer's disease. In general, the loss of higher cortical functions affects the individual's ability to respond to stresses and functional demands, while depression in Alzheimer's patients has been reported to be between 15% and 55% (Liston, 1979; Reifler, Larson & Hanley, 1982).

Reisberg (1983, p. 181) and Cohen et al., (1984) have attempted to define stage-specific concerns and psychological processes. The mild subjective symptomatology of the early phases is presumably accompanied by bewilderment and anxiety. Questions appear about one's future (What is going to happen next?), guilt (What did I do to deserve this?), and fears about changes in relationships (How do others perceive me?) and activities (What will I be able to continue doing?). At the early confusional phase, when the diagnosis is generally first made, the primary defenses are often seen as avoidance and denial. It is unclear whether the denial of specific problems represents a psychological defense (in the traditional sense of disavowal of unpleasant reality) or a lack of insight due to deficits in information processing. At this phase, characteristic differences in defensive reactions according to patient perceptions or past personality styles would be expected to occur; however, they have not yet been systematically described.

The incidence of depression is highest when the disease has progressed to moderate cognitive decline. It is not clear how much this is a result of mourning the loss of past abilities along with seeing a decrease in one's confidence and an increase in dependent needs, and how much is caused by disease-induced neurotransmitter changes influencing mood. As further deterioration occurs, agitation is often seen due to an inability to negotiate environmental stresses. Direct expression of needs or wishes via problem behaviors may result from difficulties in verbal expressiveness and judgment.

In the late-dementia phase, when verbal communicative abilities are generally lost, agitation, pacing, screaming, crying, perseveration, incontinence, or other regressive behaviors are often a communication of distress. The commonly used analogy with preverbal infants seems to apply most to this phase in terms of somatic and nonverbal communication patterns, care needs, dependency, and stimulus-bound responses. In such cases, medications without behavioral interventions do not always decrease the problem behaviors.

Delusional or paranoid ideation is often seen, and does not seem restricted to the late phases of the illness as suggested in some staging systems. Such symptoms may well represent an adaptive suspiciousness toward a progressively unfamiliar world or an attempt to provide a personal explanation for one's condition. Alternatively, subcortical neural sites of degeneration may also account for the rise in psychotic ideation and explain the relatively good symptomatic response to antipsychotic medication for a number of patients.

These proposed stage-specific concerns and psychological processes are actually highly variable as exemplified in the following examples of two cases which were first seen in the early-dementia phase of the illness and have progressed to a moderate-dementia phase.

Case 1. A 69-year-old college professor was noticing increasing difficulty teaching, having to use "crib sheets" (outlines) to help himself understand the materials that he passed out to his students. He was seen as a good natured, pollyanna-like, eccentric who prided himself on his patience and ability to persist until he completed a task. He demonstrated no denial of problems. Upon learning about his diagnosis from his internist, he began to keep an elaborate note-reminder system, retired early, and set up a rigid schedule for himself to organize his life by going to his office 7 days a week. He talked of his fascination with the process of memory, joking that his memory was second to none—none came first and his came second. He also described his memory as a ticker-tape machine—he simply had to wait long enough for the memory he wanted to flash by so he could grab it. He was able to plan for his needs through supportive psychotherapy sessions. During this phase of his illness, he showed an exaggeration of a premorbid personality style, with no evident shift in mood or personality characteristics.

Case 2. A 67-year-old teacher had increasing difficulties due to her memory problems and difficulty comprehending reading. Sometime after her performance began to decline, she began drinking heavily and refused to socialize. She was a socially isolated and critical woman with no children. Her husband had developed a life which was largely independent from hers. Her primary identification was her work. Her past history and quality of object relations suggested long-standing conflicts and a chronic sense of dissatisfaction with her life. She was forced by her husband and boss to have an evaluation, although she denied any problems. She showed depressive features, and as she became increasingly aware of disabilities, she responded by developing persecutory paranoid symptoms involving her husband and co-workers. She was seen for supportive psychotherapy and medication management. Persistent cognitive impairment was noted after improvement in depressive and paranoid symptoms and cessation of alcohol. She continues to show fears about her declining functional capabilities.

These examples demonstrate that although many cases may fit the conceptual framework of a stage-specific reaction pattern, there is also considerable variability, which can be predicted in part from the premorbid personality, education, prior work, relationships, adaptive responses, attitudes, motivation, and current level of understanding. The victims of Alzheimer's disease can be viewed as individuals with increasingly limited resources, who must come to terms with their degenerative disease and work through unresolved personal issues, generally in their own characteristic reaction patterns.

FAMILY AND CAREGIVER REACTIONS TO ALZHEIMER'S DISEASE

The family, which generally provides care for the Alzheimer's patient, is under an increasingly taxing burden throughout the progression of the disease. Although reactions and adjustments differ among families, several typical reactions have been described and seem to be intensified as the disability progresses (Brody, 1985).

Many problems that families demonstrate reflect insufficient knowledge about the disease. The lack of information can affect the quality of the coping skills and problem-solving behaviors of the caregiver, and will be reflected in the level of perceived stress as well as in the quality of care (Cohen et al., 1984; Levine, Dastoor, & Gendron, 1983). This has led to an educational family therapy approach in which caregivers are provided information to assist in problem solving and to offer support (Mace & Rabins, 1981; Zarit & Zarit, 1982).

In many families, defenses against the stress of overwhelming demands and unwanted life change create interpersonal crises. Often the stresses on the family lead to a disturbance in the family homeostasis. Long-standing conflictual issues which had existed between family members may resurface. Competitiveness or maladaptive coalitions within the family can emerge and lead to difficulties in decision making or care. In many instances, the problems of "role reversal" (children become the parents to their own parent) lead to pathological identifications with the parents or reenactments of one's own perceived childhood situation. Over-involvement, disengagement, or parent abuse are sometimes seen, and excessive guilt may be experienced when one cannot perform as an "adequate parent." Family members may even feel responsible for eliciting the patient's pathological behaviors and can experience intense feelings of guilt or depression. Under such conditions, they often need to be in treatment. In some cases, family therapy may be the treatment of choice.

Nonspecific reactions to the disorder are also seen. There is a frequent identification with the victim by other family members, characterized by fears of inheriting Alzheimer's disease. There is a tendency to deny the diagnosis for this and other reasons, to go from doctor to doctor, or to maintain unreasonable expectations of and demands on the victim. Denial is a common reaction which helps defend the family against their sense of hopelessness, but it makes realistic planning and treatment difficult. The denial must be addressed if any assistance is to be provided. Negative feelings by family members are often engendered by the irritating behaviors of the victim, or by the degree of sacrifice that caregiving requires. Expression of these feelings and assistance in working out alternative coping mechanisms are necessary in order to avoid acting out hostile feelings against the patient or developing stress-related adjustment reactions. Supportive therapy from the psychiatrist or other professional caregivers, or involvement in self-help groups or mutual support groups, may be especially useful in dealing with these problems. The intensity of service needed is dictated by the severity of the family disturbance.

The reactions of professional caregivers to various patient behaviors, as in institutional settings, may sometimes resemble the responses of family members. Psychiatric consultative services are often needed to help educate the staff to the clinical course and management of the patient, and to assist the staff in understanding the dynamics behind behavioral problems. When ongoing liaison is possible, the consultant can also help the staff deal with their frustrations in trying to cope with difficult situations, and can direct the treatment team in formulating appropriate management approaches.

TABLE 1
Natural History of Alzheimer's Disease: Clinical Findings
(NOTE: Variability in symptoms and test results is commonplace throughout the natural history.)

Minimal Cognitive Decline
(Recognized as incipient Alzheimer's disease only in retrospect; otherwise, in absence of progressive decline could be within normal limits of aging)

Concentration	Good; no deficit in calculations
Recent memory	No functional decrement but complains of forgetting familiar names or where one placed objects
Past memory	No functional decrement
Orientation	Fully oriented; no errors on mental status exams
Praxis	Normal
Self-care	Normal
Language/speech	Average
Visuospatial skills	Average
Complex/new tasks	No performance difficulties
"Personality"	No change; Possible performance anxiety
EEG	Normal
CAT scan	Normal

Early Cognitive Decline

Concentration	Mild deficit; often see errors on serial calculations
Recent memory	Decreased; name recall deficits and misplacing items become noticeable to others; often cannot recall a book passage or recent event; mild functional decrement present
Past memory	Possible deficits in recall of distant personal life events
Orientation	Generally oriented; often no errors on mental status exams
Praxis	Normal or may be variably affected
Self-care	Normal
Language/speech	Word finding problems; poor word-list generation and anomia begin
Visuospatial skills	Topographic disorientation; may get lost in unfamiliar settings; poor constructions on tests
Complex/new tasks	Decreased performance in demanding employment settings
"Personality"	Variable changes; apathy, depression, irritability
EEG	Normal
CAT scan	Normal

Moderate Cognitive Decline

Concentration	Moderate deficits; acalculia is evident on serial calculations or has difficulty counting backwards
Recent memory	Poor; poor knowledge of current and recent events
Past memory	Skeleton of past history is intact but fine details may be lost

Orientation | Frequent mistakes on orientation, but generally still oriented to date and familiar persons
Praxis | Ideomotor apraxia; difficulty handling marketing, finances, hobbies
Self-care | ADL still possible, but may require assistance in choosing clothing, needs coaxing to bathe, etc.
Language/speech | Repetitive; limited vocabulary and sentence structure; moderate language impairment may be present
Visuospatial skills | Poor construction; spatial disorientation but usually able to travel to familiar locations
Complex/new tasks | Decreased abilities; performance anxiety evident and withdraws from challenging situations
"Personality" | Variable changes; denial is often the dominant defense; indifference and apathy
EEG | Slowing of background rhythm
CAT scan | Normal or ventricular dilatation and sulcal enlargement

Severe Cognitive Decline (Dementia Phase)

Concentration | Severely deteriorated; if engagable, would have difficulty counting to 10
Recent memory | Severely deteriorated; largely unaware of all recent events and experiences
Past memory | Severely deteriorated
Orientation | Severely deteriorated; unaware of surroundings, season, etc.; may forget spouse
Praxis | Severe ideomotor apraxia (unable to use eating utensils, handle mechanics of toileting, etc.)

Self-care	Requires assistance in all spheres; develops periodic or total urinary and fecal incontinence
Language/speech	Total fluent aphasia; speech not intelligible
Visuospatial skills and motoric changes	Agraphia, limb rigidity, flexion posture; generalized and cortical neurologic signs are often present
Complex/new tasks	Unable to perform tasks
"Personality"	Variable changes; delusional behavior, obsessive symptoms and repetition; agitation/anxiety; abulia
EEG	Diffusely slow
CAT scan	Ventricular dilatation and sulcal enlargement

Adapted from Reisberg et al. (1982), Shamoian (1984), and Cummings and Benson (1983).

REFERENCES

Brody, E. (1985). The Kent lecture. *The Gerontologist, 25*(1), 19–29.

Cohen, D., Kennedy, G., & Eisdorfer, C. (1984). Phases of change in the patient with Alzheimer's dementia: A conceptual dimension of defining health care management. *Journal of the American Geriatrics Society, 32*(1), 11–15.

Crook, T., Bartus, R.T., Ferris, S.H., Whitehouse, P., Cohen, G.D., & Gershon, S. (1986). Age-associated memory impairment: Proposed diagnostic criteria and measures of clinical change—Report of a National Institute of Mental Health work group. *Developmental Neuropsychology, 2*(4), 261–276.

Cummings, J.L., & Benson, F.D. (1983). *Dementia: A clinical approach.* Boston: Butterworth.

Kahn, R.L., Goldfarb, A.I., Pollack, M., & Peck, A. (1960). Brief objective measures for the determination of mental status of the aged. *American Journal of Psychiatry, 117*, 326–328.

Kahn, R.L., & Miller, N.E. (1978). Assessment of altered brain function in the aged. In M. Storandt, E.C. Siegler, & N.F. Elias (Eds.), *The clinical psychology of aging.* New York: Plenum Press.

Kral, V. (1967). *Senescent forgetfulness: Benign and malignant. Canadian Medical Association Journal, 86*, 257–260.

Levine, N., Dastoor, D.P., & Gendron, C.E. (1983). Coping with dementia. *American Geriatrics Society, 31*(1), 12–18.

Liston, E.H. (1979). Clinical findings in presenile dementia: A report of 50 cases. *Journal of Nervous and Mental Diseases, 167*, 337–342.

McHugh, P.R., & Folstein, M.F. (1975). Psychiatric symptoms of Huntington's chorea: A clinical and phenomenologic study. In F. Benson & D. Blumer (Eds.), *Psychiatric aspects of neurological disease*. New York: Grune & Stratton.

Mace, N.L., & Rabins, P.V. (1981). *The 36-hour day: A family guide to caring for persons with Alzheimer's disease, related dementing illnesses, and memory loss in later life.* Baltimore: John's Hopkins University Press.

Marco, L., & Randels, P.M. (1984). Neurobiology of cognitive deterioration. In W.E. Kelly (Ed.), *Alzheimer's disease and related disorders: Research and management.* Springfield, IL: Charles C Thomas.

Reifler, B., Larson, E., & Hanley, R. (1982). Coexistence of cognitive impairment and depression in geriatric outpatients. *American Journal of Psychiatry, 139*(5), 623–626.

Reisberg, B., Ferris, S., De Leon, M., & Crook, T. (1982). The global deterioration scale for assessment of primary degenerative dementia. *American Journal of Psychiatry, 139*(9), 1136–1139.

Reisberg, B. (Ed.) (1983). *Alzheimer's disease: The standard reference.* New York: Free Press.

Rosen, W.G., Mohs, R.C., & Davis, K.L. (1984). A new rating scale for Alzheimer's disease. *American Journal of Psychiatry, 141*(11), 1356–1364.

Shamoian, C.A. (1984). *Biology and treatment of dementia in the elderly.* Washington, DC: American Psychiatric Press.

Wechsler, D. (1944). *The measurement of adult intelligence.* Baltimore: Williams & Wilkins.

Wells, C. (1979). Pseudodementia. *American Journal of Psychiatry, 136*, 895–900.

Zarit, S., & Zarit, J. (1982). Families under stress: Interventions for caregivers of senile dementia patients. *Psychotherapy Theory, Research, and Practice, 19*(4), 461–471.

Zarit, S., & Orr, Z.N. (1983). *Working with families of dementia victims: A treatment manual.* Washington, DC: Administration on Aging, Grant No. 90-At-2167.

3

DIAGNOSIS

The clinical diagnosis of Alzheimer's disease is based primarily on the clinical presentation and is made by a process of exclusion; a definitive diagnosis is determined by examining brain tissue (on autopsy) in combination with the prior clinical picture (American Psychiatric Association, 1987). No unequivocal diagnostic clinical or laboratory tests exist. However, any patient suspected of having a dementing illness should have a comprehensive assessment including general medical and psychiatric histories. In addition, because many patients have reversible dementias, neurologic, psychiatric and general medical clinical examinations as well as basic neuropsychological tests and laboratory studies should be conducted. Assessment of the functional capacity of the patient and an in-depth evaluation of the family and/or support systems are critical. At times, a diagnosis cannot be made immediately, and the patient must be seen more than just once. An accurate diagnosis is critical since it provides the framework for the treatment of the behavioral and psychiatric problems which are usually the major manifestations of the illness during the early and middle stages of the disorder.

GENERAL MEDICAL AND PSYCHIATRIC HISTORIES

A comprehensive history should be obtained from the patient and complemented with information from a family member or caregiver. Especially in later stages of the illness, the family member or caregiver will likely be the major or only source of clinical history, since the patient will not be able to cooperate. The history should be supplemented with discussions with treating physicians and records of prior evaluations, previous and present treatments and past hospitalizations, a comprehensive review of body systems, a review of all medications (prescribed and nonprescribed), as well as a history of alcohol use.

An assessment of changes of personality, social behavior, physical and functional abilities, eating habits and sleep patterns should be obtained, along with the presence or absence of hallucinations, delusions and suicidal ideation. Changes in motor behavior, affect and perception should be assessed, with a focus on the nature, intensity and progression of the reported symptoms. The history of a patient with Alzheimer's disease primarily reveals impaired cognitive functions and activities of daily living, mood fluctuations, and presence of delusions, illusions, and hallucinations usually in the more advanced stages of the illness (Blass, 1982). "Common complaints of patients or families include: forgetfulness about appointments or errands; inability to find the way to an accustomed destination; inability to use money and instruments of daily living such as a telephone; deterioration in work or homemaking performance; difficulty adapting to changes in the workplace; difficulties in dressing, reading and writing; and inability to recognize previously familiar individuals" (McKhann et al., 1984).

GENERAL MEDICAL ASSESSMENT

A comprehensive general medical and neurological clinical examination is required to rule out other causes of dementia.

Physical illnesses are known to aggravate the course of Alzheimer's disease (Besdine, 1982). Studies have reported that 50% of patients with Alzheimer's disease have treatable illnesses or symptoms. Every effort must be made to identify and appropriately treat underlying medical illnesses which, if untreated, may induce a superimposed state of delirium (Wells, 1978). Many prescribed and nonprescribed medications as well as physiological phenomena such as pain are notorious inducers of delirium (Besdine, 1982).

A complete neurological examination is critical to exclude neurological disorders presenting with a dementia. This examination should assess, for example, the cranial nerves, muscle tone, reflexes, coordination, and gait. Snout reflex, jaw jerk, rigidity or myoclonus are not infrequently encountered in the early stages of Alzheimer's disease (McKhann et al., 1984).

PSYCHIATRIC ASSESSMENT

This includes a comprehensive personal and psychiatric history with a focus on the mental status of the patient. Information pertaining to the mental status should be collected both formally and informally with a focus on mood, state of consciousness, speech, thought content, motoric activity, and general cognition.

An assessment, which may require follow-up evaluations, will assist in ruling out psychiatric disorders such as depression, catatonia, and drug toxicity which may mimic or induce dementia. The cognitive assessment evaluates "orientation, registration, attention, calculation, recent recall, naming, repeating, understanding, reading, writing, and ability to draw or copy " (McKhann et al., 1984).

A variety of quantitative scales are available to evaluate cognitive and personal functioning. The following scales can be found in the Appendix to this report: for cognitive functions, the Mini Mental State Exam (Folstein, Folstein & McHugh, 1975); for clinical symptoms and social functions, the Blessed Dementia Scale (Blessed, Tomlinson & Roth, 1968) and the Dementia Behavior Scale (Haycox, 1984); for multi-infarct dementia, the Hachinski Scale (Hachinski, Lassen & Marshall, 1974); and for depression, the Geriatric Depression Scale (Yesavage et al., 1983).

NEUROPSYCHOLOGICAL TESTING

Neuropsychological tests are helpful, not only in providing data confirming the diagnosis of dementia, but also in assessing the intellectual strengths still intact. These tests are important "for determining patterns of impairment, for assessing changes in impairment over time and after drug treatment or rehabilitation, and for establishing correlations of abnormal performance with laboratory and neuropathologic examinations" (McKhann et al., 1984). Assessment of cognitive impairment is complex. The clinician must determine which cognitive functions are to be evaluated. Furthermore, there is no general agreement on which specific tests best assess specific cognitive impairment. Neuropsychological functions frequently assessed are listed in Table 2.

TABLE 2
Neuropsychological Functions to Be Assessed

Attention/Concentration
Language Function
    Spoken language
    Comprehension
    Repetition
    Naming
    Reading/writing
Thought Processes
    Organization
    Content
    Abstraction
Information
Memory (Verbal and Nonverbal)
    New learning
    Delayed recall
    Recognition
    Recall of early life events
Specific Intellectual Functions
    Visuoconstructive
    Visuospatial
    Stereognosis
Nonspecific Functions
    Orientation
    Trailmaking

DIAGNOSTIC CRITERIA AND DIAGNOSTIC TESTS

The diagnosis of Alzheimer's disease should be made after comprehensive general medical, neurological and psychiatric evaluations have ruled out the other causes of dementia (Larson et al., 1986). Even with an exhaustive and comprehensive assessment, the number of false positive diagnoses of Alzheimer's disease, as determined at autopsy, remains high. Refinements of neuropsychological testing and the more recent experimental brain imaging techniques may well increase our diagnostic accuracy. However, until more reliable correlations with laboratory findings are established, the diagnosis of Alzheimer's disease will continue to be made clinically. One useful guideline to clinicians has been proposed by the Workgroup on Diagnosing Alzheimer's Disease, under the auspices of the Department of Health and Human Services Task Force on Alzheimer's disease (McKhann et al., 1984) and is summarized in Table 3.

TABLE 3
Suggested Criteria for Clinical Diagnosis of Alzheimer's Disease

The criteria for the clinical diagnosis of probable Alzheimer's disease include:

Dementia established by clinical examination and documented by the Mini-Mental Scale, Blessed Dementia Scale, or some similar examination, and possibly confirmed by neuropsychological tests;
Deficits in two or more areas of cognition; progressive worsening of memory and other cognitive functions
No disturbance of consciousness;
Onset between ages 40 and 90, most often after age 65; and
Absence of systemic disorders or other brain diseases that in and of themselves could account for the progressive deficits in memory cognition.

The diagnosis of probable Alzheimer's disease is supported by:

Progressive deterioration of specific cognitive functions such as
   language (aphasia), motor skills (apraxia), and perception
   (agnosia);
Impaired activities of daily living and altered patterns of behavior;
Family history of similar disorders, particularly if confirmed
   neuropathologically; and
Laboratory results of:
   normal lumbar puncture as evaluated by standard techniques,
   normal pattern or nonspecific changes in EEG, such as in-
      creased slow wave activity, and
   evidence of cerebral atrophy on CT with progression documented
      by serial observation.

Other clinical features consistent with the diagnosis of probable
Alzheimer's disease, after exclusion of causes of dementia other
than Alzheimer's disease, include:

Plateaus in the course of progression of the illness;
Associated symptoms such as depression, insomnia, incontinence,
   delusions, illusions, hallucinations, catastrophic verbal, emotional, or physical outbursts, sexual disorders, and weight loss;
Other neurological abnormalities in some patients, especially with
   more advanced disease and including motor signs such as increased muscle tone, myoclonus, or gait disorder;
Seizures in advanced disease; and
CT normal for age.

Features that make the diagnosis of probable Alzheimer's
disease uncertain or unlikely include:

Sudden apoplectic onset;
Focal neurologic findings such as hemiparesis, sensory loss, visual
   field deficits, and incoordination early in the course of the
   illness; and

Seizures or gait disturbances at the onset or very early in the course of the illness.

Clinical diagnosis of possible Alzheimer's disease:

May be made on the basis of the dementia syndrome in the absence of other neurologic, psychiatric, or systemic disorders sufficient to cause dementia, and in the presence of variations in the onset, in the presentation, or in the clinical course;

May be made in the presence of a second systemic or brain disorder sufficient to produce dementia which is not considered to be the cause of the dementia; and

Should be used in research studies when a single, gradually progressive severe cognitive deficit is identified in the absence of other identifiable cause.

Criteria for diagnosis of definite Alzheimer's disease are:

The clinical criteria for probable Alzheimer's disease, and
Histopathologic evidence obtained from a biopsy or autopsy.

Classification of Alzheimer's disease for research purposes should specify features that may differentiate subtypes of the disorder, such as:

Familial occurrence,
Onset before age of 65
Presence of trisomy-21, and
Coexistence of other relevant conditions such as Parkinson's disease.

Adapted from McKhann et al. (1984).

A subsequent guide to tests for the Differential Diagnosis of Dementing Disorders in general was developed at the 1987 National Institutes of Health Consensus Development Conference on this topic. This guide is shown in Table 4.

TABLE 4
Tests for the Differential Diagnosis of Dementing Disorders

The best diagnostic test is a careful history and physical and mental status examination.

The laboratory tests that are used should be individualized based on the history and physical and mental status examination. Over-testing may expose the patient to discomfort, inconvenience, excess costs, and the likelihood of false positive tests that may lead to additional unnecessary testing. Undertesting also has hazards, for example, in elderly persons, where medical disease may have nonspecific presentations such as dementia.

All patients with new onset of dementia should have several basic and standard diagnostic studies, with modifications to be made according to individual circumstances:

1. Complete blood count
2. Electrolyte panel
3. Screening metabolic panel
4. Thyroid function studies
5. Vitamin B_{12} and folate levels
6. Tests for syphilis and, depending on history, for human immunodeficiency antibodies
7. Urinalysis
8. Electrocardiogram
9. Chest x-ray

Most of the readily reversible metabolic, endocrine, deficiency, and infectious states, whether causative or complicating, will be revealed by these simple investigations when combined with history and physical examination.

Other ancillary studies are appropriate in certain common situations:

1. Computed tomography of the brain (without contrast) is appropriate in the presence of history suggestive of a mass, or focal neurologic signs, or in dementia of brief duration. Unless such diagnosis is obvious on first contact, computed tomography should be done.
2. All medications that are not absolutely necessary should be discontinued.
3. Electroencephalograms are appropriate for patients with altered consciousness or suspected seizure, depending on the clinical circumstances.
4. Formal psychiatric assessment is desirable when depression is suspected.
5. Inpatient hospitalization should be considered when the history is unclear, if the patient is suicidal, when an acute deterioration has occurred without apparent cause, or if the social situation precludes adequate observation.
6. Neuropsychological evaluation is appropriate (a) to obtain baseline information against which to measure change in cases in which diagnosis is in doubt, (b) before and following treatment, (c) in cases of exceptionally bright individuals suspected of early dementia, (d) in cases of ambiguous imaging findings that require elucidation, (e) to help distinguish dementia from depression and delirium, and (f) to provide additional information about the extent and nature of impairment following focal or multifocal brain injury.
7. Speech and language analysis can be very helpful. In some patients, complex language disorders can simulate dementia; in others, the skillful speech pathologist can help the patient and family to communicate better.

The role of other studies is controversial, and firm rules for their routine use are not appropriate. Undue weight should not be placed on isolated laboratory findings unless they are consistent with previous clinical information. Examples of these other studies include the following:

1. Magnetic resonance imaging is more sensitive than computer tomography for detection of small infarcts, mass lesions, atrophy of the brainstem, and other subcortical structures; it also may clarify ambiguous computed tomography findings. Inexperienced interpreters may make too much of ambiguous or nonspecific findings on magnetic resonance imaging.
2. Regional cerebral blood flow and metabolism measurements (positron emission tomography and single photon emission computed tomography) are research techniques that have no proven *routine* clinical value at the present time. Their value in predicting Huntington's and Alzheimer's disease in individuals at risk is under investigation.
3. Lumbar puncture is not routinely required in the initial evaluation of dementia. It should be performed when other clinical findings suggest an active infection or vasculitis. At present, cerebrospinal fluid markers for Alzheimer's disease are not sufficiently well developed to justify routine lumbar puncture.
4. Electrophysiological techniques such as event-related potentials that are recorded using special electroencephalographic techniques are not recommended for routine use.
5. Brain biopsy for nontumorous and noninfectious diseases rarely is justified except in a small number of unusual clinical situations.
6. Biological markers for progressive degenerative dementing disease are still in the investigative stage. Although some give promise, they are not ready for widespread or routine use.
7. Significant major findings have been made on the molecular genetics of conditions like Huntington's and Alzheimer's diseases, but these findings have restricted usefulness at present.
8. Carotid ultrasound is of no value except sometimes in the search for the cause of infarcts.

From the National Institutes of Health Consensus Development Statement, 1987.

DIFFERENTIAL DIAGNOSIS OF ALZHEIMER'S DISEASE

The diagnosis of Alzheimer's disease can be confounded by a variety of dementias and dementia-like syndromes. These include the primary and secondary causes of dementia and certain psychiatric disorders, many of which have specific and nonspecific treatments available (Wells, 1982). The rate of progression of a number of these other dementias can be attenuated or even arrested once treatment is instituted; in fact, the observable cognitive deficits due to the secondary causes of dementia may be reversible.

Age-Associated Memory Impairment

Many elderly patients complain of symptoms, especially memory difficulties, which are similar to those found in Alzheimer's disease (Crook et al., 1986; Kral, 1978). However, these patients do not have the typical history of a progressive deterioration but continue to function socially and to care for themselves. The cognitive deficit has been considered by various investigators to be a variant of normal aging and these patients presumably do not eventually become demented. The cognitive problems consist of forgetting specific dates and names. Unlike the memory impairment in Alzheimer's patients, this deficit is inconsistent, and frequently within a short period of time the forgotten memory is recalled. Neuropsychological testing reveals only mild deficits, which may progress only slightly over the years (Kral, 1978). Since this phenomenon has been viewed as a variant of normal aging, it is generally not considered to be pathological and must be differentiated from the latter conditions. This age-associated memory impairment may encompass the concept of "benign senescent forgetfulness" (Kral, 1978).

Pseudodementia of Psychiatric Etiology

Approximately 10–12% of patients diagnosed as being demented are not, in fact, but have an underlying psychiatric disorder which presents with cognitive dysfunctions. Significant depressive symptomatology is common, with prevalence rates ranging from 10% to 50% (Gershon & Herman, 1982). Moreover, in the elderly, physical illness, which is common in this age group, is intimately related to depression. Of the elderly who have general medical illnesses, 30–50% are afflicted with an affective disorder (Dovenmuehle & Verwoerdt, 1962). Approximately 75–80% of patients with a depression have a completely reversible psychiatric illness when appropriately treated. Pseudodemented patients not infrequently complain of poor memory, including disorientation to time and place and impaired short-term memory. They complain also of difficulty in comprehending questions and instructions, poor concentration, and being easily distracted (Wells, 1979). These patients, in addition, usually have the typical signs and symptoms of depression including dysphoria, anxiety, agitation, guilt, anorexia, decreased libido, insomnia, weight loss, etc. In the elderly depressed patient, somatic preoccupation and complaints are common.

Pseudodementia may be difficult to differentiate clinically from a true dementia. However, the onset of a pseudodementia is usually abrupt, whereas that of a true dementia is gradual. The pseudodemented patient will often have disturbances in sleep, appetite, and energy, and not infrequently will have had a prior history of episodes of depression. Moreover these patients can be quite verbal and aware of their cognitive deficits and disabilities, whereas patients with Alzheimer's disease often deny their cognitive difficulties. When given an appropriate trial of antidepressants, the cognitive deficits of the pseudodemented patient disappear with the amelioration of the underlying depression. Treatment of patients with Alzheimer's disease with antidepressants, in the absence of depression, will not improve cognitive functions and in fact may accentuate them.

Pseudodementia is not restricted to depression, but can occur in other psychiatric conditions such as schizophrenia (Lishman, 1978). A history of the illness and its course clearly differentiates it from Alzheimer's disease. Indeed, elderly chronic schizophrenics may also be afflicted with Alzheimer's disease. The latter can be aggravated by the anticholinergic side effects of the antipsychotic drugs used for treating the schizophrenic process. In chronic schizophrenics, dementia symptoms should not automatically be assumed to be secondary to the psychiatric illness. In fact, they often may be reversible once the etiology is identified and effectively treated.

Catatonic schizophrenics can, because of their mutism and abnormal behavior, be misconstrued as being demented. Because of the rarity of this condition and its history, the differential diagnosis should not present a problem.

Mania in the elderly can present with cognitive dysfunction, which can easily be misconstrued as due to Alzheimer's disease. With effective treatment of the mania these deficits will disappear. Usually there is a history of mania or depression which will assist in the diagnosis.

Anxiety is a symptom common to a variety of psychiatric and nonpsychiatric illnesses. Not uncommonly the elderly anxious individual will have great difficulty in concentrating, focusing on the task, and responding to questions appropriately. These individuals can easily be misdiagnosed as early-stage Alzheimer's disease. In many patients, this is the manner in which Alzheimer's disease begins, but in the truly nondemented anxious person, appropriate treatment will clarify the issue.

Drug-Induced Encephalopathy

The elderly ingest a variety of different medications—prescribed and nonprescribed (Bozzetti & MacMurry, 1977; Lamy, 1981). Drugs and/or drug-drug interactions may lead to a dementia-like syndrome or a toxic confusional state. Any differential diagnosis of a dementia must include the possibility of a drug(s)-induced phenomenon. For example, the elderly patient ingesting anticholinergic drugs can present a clinical picture of disorientation, difficulty in concentration, poor recent memory, etc., which can easily be misconstrued as the beginnings of Alzheimer's disease. Whenever possible, the number of medications prescribed to patients should be kept to a minimum and patients suspected of a dementia should have all medications except life-sustaining drugs discontinued. This will assist in making the appropriate diagnosis, and more often than not the symptoms will be associated, in time, with the ingestion of medications.

Even if the patient is afflicted with Alzheimer's disease, potentially dementing drugs should be discontinued or dosages kept to a minimum to abate the impact of the dementia.

Multi-Infarct Dementia

Multi-infarct dementias alone or in combination with Alzheimer's disease account for approximately 15–30% of the dementias (Blass, 1982). Patients with multi-infarct dementia typically have numerous small strokes which result primarily in a dementia rather than motoric deficiencies. Larger strokes are more likely to be associated with more apparent motoric manifestations. The progression of the illness is typically stepwise, with periods of relative stability in between each episode. Not infrequently, each episode is marked by a transient ischemic attack. Eventually these patients develop overt signs of cerebral, cardiac or peripheral vascular disease. The diagnosis, which may be made by history and physical examination, can also be confirmed by the use of the Hachinski scale (Hachinski et al., 1974) (see Appendix). Frequently the history of these patients will reveal, in addition to the stepwise deterioration, an abrupt onset, nocturnal confusion, a relative preservation of the personality, a history of hypertension and strokes, and focal neurological signs and symptoms. However, not all patients will manifest a stepwise deterioration. The incidence of multi-infarct dementia peaks at the ages of 40–60 years and occurs more frequently in men than in women (Gershon & Herman, 1982). In Alzheimer's disease, however, dementia increases gradually in incidence with advancing age and is more common in women than in men (Gershon & Herman, 1982). Patients with multi-infarct dementia are known to benefit from early therapeutic intervention for the control of hypertension, arrhythmias, and diabetes mellitus.

Normal Pressure Hydrocephalus

The syndrome of normal pressure hydrocephalus (NPH), first described by Hakim and Adams (1965), consists of a triad of clinical manifestations: gait disturbance, which is often the presenting symptom; progressive dementia; and eventually urinary incontinence. Two types of NPH have been described: The first is secondary to head trauma, subarachnoid hemorrhage, or meningitis. The second is the idiopathic type with an insidious onset and progressive course. Surgical insertion of a shunt, which is rarely performed, often abates the triad of symptoms. Patients with primarily gait disturbance are considered the best surgical candidates (Shenkin et al., 1973).

The early behavior changes of NPH may be the same as those of Alzheimer's disease, or typical of frontal lobe disease, and include apathy, irritability and socially unacceptable behavior. There may be alternating episodes of lethargy and confusion, urinary frequency, and minimal cognitive deficits. Reflex abnormalities including Babinski's sign are frequently present. This clinical picture may remain stable for months, but more often than not it progresses over a period of weeks to months to a state in which the patient has difficulty with balance and is mute, paranoid or depressed, incontinent and severely demented (Strub & Black, 1981). NPH accounts for up to 5% of the dementias (Strub & Black, 1981).

Brain Tumors

Tumors of the temporal and frontal lobes are known to produce a number of mental changes. Dementia, mental dullness, amnesia, confusion, apathy, euphoria, irritability and inappropriate social behavior are common (Strub & Black, 1981). Though brain tumors can mimic Alzheimer's disease, most of them can be distinguished by a focal neurological abnormality or a clouding of consciousness. They may be responsible for 3–10% of the reported dementias (Strub & Black, 1981).

Dementia and Carcinoma

Many patients with carcinoma of an organ system other than the central nervous system may manifest a dementia. Dementia is more common in those patients who have central nervous system involvement. The symptoms of dementia are usually those associated with intellectual deterioration and failure of memory (Strub & Black, 1981).

Subdural Hematomas

Chronic subdural hematomas are common in the elderly, even without a history of brain trauma (Strub & Black, 1981). Usually there are focal neurological abnormalities or fluctuating states of consciousness. Not infrequently patients may present with sudden mental or personality changes. A subdural hematoma must be ruled out in these patients.

Infections and Inflammatory Diseases

Chronic meningitis due to tuberculosis, cryptococcosis and fungi can present with memory difficulty, headache, malaise, and visual blurring (Lishman, 1978; Strub & Black, 1981). In some of these infections such as cryptococcosis, the patient may have a 1- or 2-year history of gradual mental deterioration. This is not unlike the presentation of Alzheimer's disease. Spinal fluid examination will assist in the diagnosis.

Neurosyphilis (general paresis) may present with changes in personality associated with frontal lobe atrophy and dementia symptoms. In the late stages of the illness there is an accentuated failure of memory, aphasia, apraxia and agnosia (Lishman, 1978; Strub & Black, 1981). The paretic patient usually manifests tremors of the extremities, increased reflexes, dysarthria and Argyll Robertson pupils. A positive VDRL and spinal fluid examination will confirm the diagnosis.

Until recently, dementias due to infections have not been common, though syphilis may be responsible for 1–2% of the reported dementias. Acquired immune deficiency syndrome (AIDS) is changing this situation. While the frequency of AIDS dementia in older adults is not known, some data are available. One study identified 10% of AIDS positive cases to be 50 years of age or older and 2.5% to be 60 years of age or older, the predominant source of infection being from transfusions (Moss & Miles, 1987).

Metabolic Disorders

Many untreated metabolic disorders and states of vitamin deficiency may result in a dementia (Strub & Black, 1981). The longer the dementia is present, the more likely it is that the cognitive deficits will not be reversed by instituting treatment. These metabolic disorders and deficiency states should be considered in the differential diagnosis of a dementia.

Thyroid Disease

Hyperthyroidism may be characterized by confusion, anxiety, and a hyperactive state. In the elderly, this may, not infrequently, present atypically as a state of apathy, dullness and dementia which is usually more characteristic of hypothyroidism or myxedema. In the latter state, the dementia is characterized by slow thinking, decreased memory, and difficulty in abstractions. Long before the dementia appears, the typical symptoms of myxedema are noted, including weight gain, husky voice, thin hair, loss of lateral eyebrows, facial puffiness, and cold intolerance. Even with replacement therapy, permanent intellectual deficits have been reported (Haase, 1977). Thyroid disease is responsible for approximately 1–2% of the dementias.

Pituitary Diseases

Dementia may be associated with disease of the pituitary gland (Strub & Black, 1981). In adrenal hyperplasia and Cushing's syndrome, mental dullness and mental impairment are common symptoms. Prior to the appearance of the dementia, the other typical signs and symptoms of excessive steroids are present.

Parathyroid Disease

Cognitive deficits are not uncommon in both hyper- and hypoparathyroidism (Strub & Black, 1981). In hyperparathyroidism, the clinical picture of a toxic confusional syndrome is common. In hypoparathyroidism, dementia may be present even in the absence of tetany. A precipitous drop of serum calcium is usually associated with toxic confusional state. Cataracts, seizures and parkinsonian symptoms are often associated with hypoparathyroidism. Irreversible intellectual deficts are not uncommon even with treatment.

Vitamin Deficiencies

Vitamin deficiencies are probably more common than suspected, especially in the malnourished elderly and alcoholics (Lishman, 1978). Niacin deficiency is characterized by confusion, disorientation, memory impairment and apathy. This treatable condition is accompanied by a peripheral neuropathy, diarrhea and a dermatitis. Vitamin B_{12} and folate deficiencies can result in dementias that resemble the early stages of Alzheimer's disease. Typically, anxiety, irritability, memory impairment, decreased concentration, and decreased libido occur prior to the hematologic abnormalities. Demented patients with a history of gastric surgery and malabsorption should be suspected of this deficiency. If the illness is long-standing it will be accompanied by irreversible neurologic and psychiatric symptoms (Strub & Black, 1981). Although the true incidence of dementia due to vitamin deficiencies is not known, these should be considered in the differential diagnosis since they are easily treated.

Dialysis Dementia

Patients who are on renal dialysis for a number of years may develop a syndrome characterized by a speech disorder, myoclonus and mental changes (Alfrey, LeGendre & Kalhny, 1976). This syndrome is the major cause of death in many of the chronic dialysis patients. Subtle personality changes are common, along with a marked speech disorder which eventually yields to mutism. Asterixis, facial grimacing, myoclonus, episodes of confusion, cognitive deficits and seizures are eventually noted. Subsequently, a chronic dementia with facial and limb weakness develops. The EEG with variable patterns is abnormal. Patients dying from this syndrome have been reported at autopsy to have high concentrations of brain aluminum.

Dementia and Alcoholism

Long-term abuse of alcohol can lead to a picture clinically indistinguishable from Alzheimer's disease. Discriminating alcoholic dementia from Alzheimer's disease is complicated by the fact that some elderly patients with Alzheimer's disease also have a history of alcohol abuse. Up to 10% of the dementias in some studies are due to alcohol, and discontinuation of the intoxicant may halt the progression of the illness. Alcohol abuse associated with thiamine deficiency, referred to as Wernicke-Korsakoff syndrome, results in mental confusion, a state of lethargy, and eventually nystagmus, opthalmoplegia, ataxia, and polyneuropathy. With appropriate treatment, recovery is usually quite rapid. The acute stage of the illness has an associated mortality rate of approximately 20%.

Degenerative Diseases

Pick's Disease. Pick's disease is clinically difficult to distinguish from Alzheimer's disease (Strub & Black, 1981). During the initial stages of Pick's disease, the patient may present with change in personality and deviant social behavior rather than cognitive dysfunctions. These patients may lack insight into their problem. Later in the course of the illness, patients with Pick's disease develop an anomic aphasia with minimal, spontaneous speech production. In the middle stages of Pick's disease there is a loss of comprehension. Perseveration and echolalia may become common. In addition, some Pick's patients have a blunted affect and eat voraciously. In the final stages of the illness, similar to Alzheimer's disease, mutism, profound dementia and flexion paraplegia appear. The onset of the illness is in the early fifties with a male to female ratio of 1 : 1. An autosomal dominant genetic pattern has been suggested. Since this is a very rare disease, the chances are 50–100 : 1 that the dementia diagnosed will be that of Alzheimer's and not Pick's disease (Terry, 1976).

Huntington's Chorea. This is a familial disease, with an autosomal dominant pattern of inheritance, characterized by mental changes and chorea (Strub & Black, 1981). It occurs usually between ages 25 and 45, with changes in social behavior and emotions, including apathy, irritability, explosive behavior and lack of motivation. Unlike Alzheimer's disease, aphasia, agnosia, apraxia and amnesia are not present as the illness progresses. In the final stages of the illness, the patient is usually severely demented. The diagnosis of this illness is based on family history and neurological findings. Huntington's Chorea may account for 4–7% of the reported dementias in some series.

Parkinson's Disease. Parkinsonism is relatively common and is characterized by rigidity, tremors and slowness of movement (Lishman, 1978; Strub & Black, 1981). Although dementia occurs in this illness, it is not a presenting symptom. Depression is common in this illness and may be part of the early presentation. Usually, as the disease progresses, dementia becomes evident and the severity of the dementia correlates with the presence of severe neurological symptoms such as rigidity and akinesia. Of patients with Parkinson's disease, 25–50% manifest an intellectual decline. Cognitive problems usually include difficulty with constructional tasks, memory deficits, decreased verbal fluency, speech perception problems, and episodes of confusion. Treatment of this illness with L-dopa does not appear to reverse the cognitive deficits (Loranger et al., 1972). Some patients treated with L-dopa may in fact develop a confusional state secondary to the drug. Some patients may present with a clinical picture of a mixed Alzheimer's and Parkinson's diseases.

Creutzfeld-Jakob Disease. This extremely rare disease is caused by a slow growing transmissible virus (Lishman, 1978; Strub & Black, 1981). The illness has its onset with vague symptoms such as depression, anxiety, and memory deficits. Neurologic signs of various tracts can be seen in combination or alone. Within six months, severe dementia, rigidity and mutism develop and death usually ensues within a year. The EEG with a typical pattern of biphasic and triphasic slow waves will assist in diagnosing the disease (Haase, 1977).

REFERENCES

Alfrey, A.C., LeGendre, G.R., & Kaehny, W.D. (1976). The dialysis encephalopathy syndrome. *New England Journal of Medicine, 294,* 184.

American Psychiatric Association. (1987). *Diagnostic and statistical manual of mental disorders* (3rd ed., rev.) (DSM-III-R). Washington, DC: APA.

Besdine, R.W., (1982). Dementia. In J.W. Rowe & R.W. Besdine (Eds.), *Health and disease in old age.* Boston: Little, Brown.

Blass, J.P. (1982). Dementia, in clinical pharmacology of symptom control. (M.M. Reidenberg, Ed.) *The Medical Clinic of North America, 66,* 1143–1160.

Blessed, G., Tomlinson, B.E., & Roth, M. (1968). The association between quantitative measures of dementia and of senile change in the cerebral grey matter of elderly subjects. *British Journal of Psychiatry, 114,* 797–811.

Bozzetti, L.P., & MacMurry, J.P. (1977). Drug misuse among the elderly: A hidden menace. *Psychiatric Annals, 7,* 95–107.

Crook, T., Bartus, R.T., Ferris, S.H., Whitehouse, P., Cohen, G.D., & Gershon, S. (1986). Age-associated memory impairment: Proposed diagnostic criteria and measures of clinical change—Report of a National Institute of Mental Health work group. *Developmental Neuropsychology, 2*(4), 261–276.

Dovenmuehle, R.H., & Verwoerdt, A. (1962). Physical illness and depressive symptoms in hospitalized cardiac patients. *Journal of the American Geriatric Society, 10,* 932.

Folstein, M., Folstein, S., & McHugh, P.R. (1975). Mini-mental state: A practical method of grading the cognitive state of patients for the clinician. *Journal of Psychiatric Research, 12,* 189–198.

Gershon, S., & Herman, S.P. (1982). The differential diagnosis of dementia. *Journal of the American Geriatric Society, 30,* S58–S66.

Haase, G.R. (1977). Diseases presenting as dementia. In C.E. Wells (Eds.), *Dementia* (pp. 27–67). Philadelphia: F.A. Davis.

Hachinski, V.C., Lassen, N.A., & Marshall, J. (1974). Multi-infarct dementia: A cause of mental deterioration in the elderly. *Lancet, 2,* 207–209.

Hakim, S., & Adams, R.D. (1965). The special clinical problems of symptomatic hydrocephalus with normal cerebrospinal fluid pressure. Observations in archospinal fluid dynamics. *Journal of Neurological Science, 2,* 307.

Haycox, J.A. (1984). The Dementia Behavior Scale. *Journal of Clinical Psychiatry, 45,* 23–24.

Kral, V.A. (1978). Benign sensescent forgetfulness. In R. Katzmann, R.D. Terry & K.L. Bick (Eds.), *Alzheimer's disease, senile dementia and related disorders.* (Aging, Vol. 7) New York: Raven Press.

Lamy, P.P. (1981). Drug prescribing for elderly. *Bulletin of the New York Academy of Medicine, 57,* 718–730.

Larson, E.B., Reifler, B.V., Sumi, S.M., et al. (1986). Diagnostic tests in the evaluation of dementia. *Archives of Internal Medicine, 146,* 1917.

Lishman, W.A. (1978). *Organic psychiatry: The psychological consequences of Cerebral Disorder.* London: Blackwell.

Loranger, A.W., Goodell, H., Lee, J.E., et al. (1972). Levodopa treatment of parkinsonism syndrome. *Archives of General Psychiatry, 26,* 163.

McKhann, G., Drachman, D., Folstein, M., et al. (1984). Clinical diagnosis of Alzheimer's disease: Report of the NINCDS-ADRDA work group under the auspices of Department of Health and Human Services Task Force on Alzheimer's disease. *Neurology, 34,* 939–944.

Moss, R.J. & Miles, S.H. (1987). AIDS and the geriatrician. *Journal of the American Geriatric Society, 35,* 460–464.

National Institutes of Health Consensus Development Statement. (1987, July 6–8). *Differential diagnosis of dementing diseases, 6*(11).

Shenkin, H.A., Greenberg, J. Bouzarth, W.F., et al. (1973). Ventricular shunting for relief of senile symptoms. *Journal of the American Medical Association, 225,* 1486.

Strub, R.L., & Black, F.W. (1981). *Organic brain syndromes: An introduction to neurobehavioral disorders.* Philadelphia: FA Davis.

Terry, R.D. (1976). Dementia. *Archives of Neurology, 33,* 1.

Wells, C.E. (1978). Chronic brain disease: An overview. *American Journal of Psychiatry 135,* 1–12.

Wells, C.E. (1979). Pseudodementia. *American Journal of Psychiatry, 136,* 895.

Wells, C.E. (1982). Treatable forms of dementia. In Isselbacher, Adams, Baunwald, et al. (Eds.), *Harrison's principles of internal medicine* (update II, pp. 221–238). New York: McGraw-Hill.

Yesavage, J.A., Brink, T.L., Rose, T.I., et al. (1983). Development and validation of a geriatric depression screening scale. A preliminary report. *Journal of Psychiatric Research, 17,* 37–49.

4

TREATMENT

When the diagnosis of Alzheimer's disease has been made, the psychiatrist may be under pressure from the patient and family to initiate some kind of treatment. Unfortunately, there is no treatment available to reverse or retard the degenerative changes of this disease. There are, however, a variety of behavioral, supportive psychotherapeutic, and psychopharmacologic approaches available that may be of help to patients, their caregivers, and their families in alleviating symptoms and enhancing coping skills at different points along the course of the disorder. A number of these approaches are discussed below. Stage of illness is a key consideration in treatment planning, since problems and capacities change greatly during the clinical course of AD. At an early stage of illness, anxiety associated with high awareness of cognitive decline may respond well to supportive psychotherapeutic intervention; at a later stage of illness, marked agitation accompanying worsening delusions may be alleviated by pharmacologic treatment. In the discussions of behavioral and psychotherapeutic approaches, this chapter focuses more on concepts, with specifics further reflected throughout the case examples in the next chapter of the report.

PSYCHOTHERAPEUTIC AND PSYCHOSOCIAL TREATMENT

With the emergence of new biological insights into the nature of various mental disorders coupled with increased familiarity in using pharmacologic agents for treatment, the role of psychotherapy has often receded into the background. Such has been the case particularly with organic mental disorders. Nonetheless, effective treatment or management of major mental illness or of brain disease like Alzheimer's, where symptoms are so strongly behavioral, is best accomplished with an integration of social, psychological, and biological approaches. A focus must be maintained on patient and family alike.

Within this integrated approach, psychotherapeutic techniques may help to alleviate anxiety and depression, which can compound an Alzheimer patient's already impaired cognitive functions. Problem behavior linked to frustration, which can give way to hostility and aggressiveness, might also be ameliorated, particularly early in the course of the disorder when the patient still retains the ability to recognize and understand the nature of the clinical changes that are occurring. The establishment of an early therapeutic alliance with the patient and with his or her family not only can lead to a high level of emotional support for the entire family, but also can facilitate earlier planning to deal with the progressive clinical course of Alzheimer's disease. There is the opportunity to coordinate continuity of care that can lead to both a better treatment/management plan for the patient and a reduction in stress level for other family members providing care. In the process, the caregiver becomes a colleague in developing the treatment plan, as formal and informal systems of care become linked as important allies in improving patient care and family support.

Children of Alzheimer patients may especially benefit from family therapy. They need to deal with their painful reactions to their parent's condition and with ambivalence about the many difficult decisions that they are required to make, such as nursing home placement. They need to deal with their fears and anxiety about troubling questions such as whether they themselves will inherit Alzheimer's disease. Often guilt or dread will prevent the family from raising these and other questions. The therapist should assume that these concerns are present and approach them with the proper tact, timing, and information.

Indeed, the prevalence of reactive depression among family members in response to a loved one victimized by Alzheimer's disease is disturbingly high, with some studies reporting as many as

80% of close caregiving relatives developing significant depressive symptomatology during the course of the patient's illness (Gallagher, 1987). The fact that the clinical state of the patient with Alzheimer's disease continues to change over time makes it all the more important that families have the opportunity for ongoing consultation, so that both patient and family can be helped to maximize coping and adjustment in the face of new decrements and stresses.

The idea of psychotherapy as a potential component of an overall treatment approach for Alzheimer's disease occasionally elicits a sense of puzzlement or even derision. These critics, however, are usually thinking of patients at an advanced stage of dementia. Countertransference can also interfere with therapists working with older patients, including those with cognitive impairment (Group for the Advancement of Psychiatry, 1971; Lewis & Johansen, 1982). It is often forgotten that all patients go through earlier stages of the disorder, where the awareness of decline can be quite traumatic. It is during the early to middle stages of the disease that the role of psychotherapy can be more easily appreciated, and where the opportunity for it to reduce stress and maximize a sense of dignity in the face of decline is most apparent. Moreover, the form of psychotherapy applied with Alzheimer patients is predominantly supportive. This is not to say that psychodynamic considerations, drawing upon psychoanalytic theory, do not apply. Indeed a psychodynamic perspective can assist efforts to understand various altered thoughts, emotions, and behaviors that Alzheimer patients may manifest.

Ego Functions and Psychological Mechanisms of Defense

Psychoanalytic investigations relevant to Alzheimer's disease date back over three quarters of a century (Brosin, 1952; Goldstein, 1939; Hollos & Ferenczi, 1925; von Bertalanffy, 1974). References to these investigations are scattered through the classical psychoanalytic literature (Hartmann, 1961) as well as in current geriatric literature (Verwoerdt, 1981), though the theoretical psychodynamics of dementia as applied to the individual patient remain obscure.

But as psychoanalysis has continued its exploration of ego psychology, psychotherapists and analysts have come to recognize the importance of ego dysfunction in demented patients.

Attention to and the ability to differentiate ego functions have changed significantly over the last 20 years. Current psychoanalytic thinking has contributed to our understanding of psychological responses used as defensive operations against anxiety and depression in Alzheimer patients (Brenner, 1982). In addition, efforts are underway to correlate certain psychodynamic aspects of ego functioning in dementia with some of the more precise measurements of cognitive change emerging from neuropsychological investigations in these subjects (Bellak, Hurvich & Gedimen, 1973; Hauser, 1978; Verwoerdt, 1981).

These investigators have described techniques in which analytically based observation or interview can be quantified. Hauser has attempted to correlate psychoanalytic ego theory with data from other areas of psychological investigation, particularly "from several theories that have dealt with self, cognitive, character, moral and interpersonal development" (Hauser, 1978). It has also been suggested (Bellak et al., 1973) that the following ego functions are testable:

reality testing
judgment
sense of reality
regulation and control of drives, affect, and impulses
object relations
thought processes
adaptive regression in the service of the ego
defensive functionings
autonomous functioning
synthetic integrated function and mastery
competence

The specific effect on the deterioration of these ego functions as the dementing process continues has not been accurately described.

Problems in reality testing, judgment, defensive functioning, thought processes, and object relations, along with the regulation and control of drives, affects, and impulses, are commonly observed when treating demented patients. From an educational point of view, observing and identifying the changing nature of these ego functions can sharpen the understanding of psychodynamic phenomena by psychiatric residents and other students of mental functioning.

Buttressing these ego functions is a major aim in providing psychotherapeutic support for Alzheimer patients, though this process has not been well developed for treating such cases. The description of unconscious awareness of organic loss as manifested in dream content dates back at least to the early 1960s (Altschuler, Barad & Goldfarb, 1963). Nathan, Rose-Itkoff and Lord (1981) looked at the nature of "loss" content in dreams in relation to brain atrophy and described a correlation. Conscious and unconscious awareness by these patients of their own deficits has also been described by Verwoerdt (1981), pointing to potential clinical benefit in dealing with psychodynamic issues surrounding loss. The effect of psychotherapy in alleviating the aggravating symptoms of depression or anxiety in Alzheimer's disease might be enhanced via this focus.

It has also been suggested that Alzheimer patients who do not manifest depressive symptomatology may be constructively using a combination of denial and suppression as psychological mechanisms of defense. As a result, they contain either their degree of awareness of impairment or the way in which they interpret their dysfunction. Moderate hyperactivity in some patients has been looked at as a euphoric defense against depression (Lewin, 1950). To the extent that denial or repression appear greatly exaggerated in response to worsening losses, anxiety that compounds cognitive difficulties is also often witnessed. This dynamic has been considered in the development of "catastrophic reactions"—states of extreme anxiety and disorganization in response to frustrating challenges (Goldstein, 1939).

Discussions of the relationship between ego, superego, and id manifestations become murky as the clinical course of Alzheimer's disease advances. Generally, ego dysfunction is considerably more apparent than superego impairment. Psychodynamic aspects of changes in judgment and self-preservative behavior have been looked at, although perceptual and memory deficits have been seen as the major influences here (Schilder, 1953). In the extremely demented state, a conservation-withdrawal phenomenon has been considered. The manifestation of Alzheimer patients at this stage making no attempt to maintain contact with reality or objects has been viewed as an outcome of both marked brain tissue changes and the conservation of limited ego resources (Engel, 1962). Those at endstage dementia have been regarded psychodynamically as experiencing a complete breakdown of the ego and its defenses with apparent reciprocal dedifferentiation of the id.

Psychotherapy of Patients with Dementia

Psychoanalytic theorists from Freud on have disagreed about the use of psychoanalysis in the treatment of the aged, let alone patients with senile dementia. Half a century ago Grotjahn (1940) published his classic psychoanalytic investigation of a 71-year-old man with senile dementia. While the patient was incapable of free associations, he could speak freely to the psychoanalyst, and the therapist demonstrated that a positive transference could be accomplished. Grotjahn saw the patient for 3 weeks, 2 hours every day "and sometimes longer," then daily during the following 4 months. During the analysis, the patient's destructive behaviors were eliminated.

The analyst sat next to the patient as they both looked out the window, the patient preferring not to use the couch. Occasionally they took walks, which were useful in the production of new material. In his paper, Grotjahn addressed the timelessness of the id. In discussing the patient's defects, which were of both recent and remote memory, Grotjahn saw certain interesting inconsistencies and parapraxes. The patient, for example, said defensively, "I do not try to remember names," but frequently substituted an obvious slip, "I try to forget names." This 5-month analysis appears to represent the only such case in the psychoanalytic literature.

Seeing Alzheimer patients five to seven times a week on an hourly basis for psychotherapy is neither practical nor considered indicated, though another point of view had been expressed about a different dementing disorder (general paresis) by Hollos and Ferenczi (1925). Briefer forms of psychotherapy were later employed by a number of investigators. Butler (1960) wrote about the application of psychotherapy to geriatric patients in an inpatient unit and described positive treatment effects in cases with cognitive defects. In general, the effectiveness of brief psychotherapy in alleviating disturbing affect and behavior in Alzheimer's disease has been well described since the early 1950s. Goldfarb, in particular, was known for such pioneering approaches. One of his techniques was to allow patients to maintain certain transference distortions in order to accomplish a feeling of increased self-esteem, through a perception of greater control in relation to the therapist. The goal was also to facilitate the generalization of this positive transference effect to other significant relationships and interactions of patients with their environments (Goldfarb & Turner, 1953). Sessions lasted 5–10 minutes weekly, usually for a maximum of eight visits, and were remarkably successful in achieving their goals. Goldfarb saw these interventions as part of a total treatment program for patients with senile dementia. His technique has been taught to and incorporated into the practice of a large number of mental health professionals.

Goldfarb focused strongly on the adverse affective and behavioral symptoms that developed in demented patients in relation to their increased dependency and the accompanying conflicts. Verwoerdt (1981) expanded the focus on defensive operations in relation to symptom formation. He has looked at the significant effects that three defensive orientations in particular have had on the clinical picture of Alzheimer patients. Specifically, he has elaborated the consequences of struggles 1) for more mastery and control, 2) to exclude the threat of perceiving cognitive impairment from awareness, and 3) to retreat from this threat with conservation of energy.

Verwoerdt has emphasized that "psychotherapy with patients who have senile dementia is an essential part of a comprehensive treatment approach; the other therapeutic components include somatic treatment, environmental manipulation, and behavior therapy."

Much remains to be explored about the optimal application of psychotherapy for Alzheimer patients. Clearly, it is not sufficient to say that the patient is demented and can benefit from psychotherapy. Stage of illness, nature of symptoms, and level of capacity for interpersonal interaction are all of high and obvious relevance, determining the appropriateness and proper timing for psychotherapy. Refinement is needed in how psychotherapy is applied to these patients in the context of an underlying brain disorder with a deteriorating course. What range of techniques can be considered, and what changes in technique might have to be adopted in the same patient over time? The role of psychotherapeutic intervention in relation to specific symptoms could be better understood. How can it be best utilized in mitigating a patient's troubled thoughts, disturbed affect, or maladaptive behavior? At the same time, the role of psychotherapy in relation to the family system as a whole in the case of Alzheimer's disease needs to be kept in mind.

Family Therapy

Despite widespread belief, it appears not to be the case that in the "good old days" spouses or children took better care of their demented spouses or parents than they do today (Brody, 1985). The myth of the ungrateful spouse or child seems to represent a projected wish that if only the family were more available, the patient's dementia could be overcome. In fact, a large majority of demented patients are cared for within the family, either directly or by surrogates.

Excellent resource books on caring for Alzheimer's disease have been developed for family members (Cohen & Eisdorfer, 1986; Mace & Rabins, 1981). Families should be encouraged and assisted in linking up with other resources as well, both to aid them in their caregiving capacity and to relieve burden. Experts on financial and legal planning, for example, are very important, given the heavy economic demands that too many families suffer—and the emotional toll from this added burden.

For family members, the burdens of care often result in depression, anger, and guilt. Despite the paucity of information on the psychodynamic processes in such situations, it seems safe to assert that the dynamics differ from family to family. Meanwhile, the psychiatric literature on family issues in AD is growing (Ory et al., 1985; Rabins, Mace & Lucas, 1982; Reifler & Wu, 1982; Teusink & Mahler, 1984).

From a more theoretical point of view, the question arises as to how the various accumulated identifications and object relationships that exist in the child or spousal caregiver undergo changes, and what results when these object losses begin to accumulate. Perhaps these are the intrapsychic phenomena that lead to the depressions that are reported so frequently in caregivers.

From a contextual family therapy perspective, the child may view the parent as one toward whom he or she has an obligation and debt. Caring for the parent would allow at least a partial payment and would entitle the child to repayment from his or her own children. Parentification of the caregiver usually does not take place only as the result of the severe dementia of the patient, but has roots earlier in the relationship. For example, the wife who "sacrifices her marriage" to take care of a demented parent may have had a disturbed marriage prior to the onset of the new stress and uses the need to help her parent as an excuse to distance herself from her spouse.

Often it is necessary to see both the demented patient and the family together in early sessions. The spouse and children who bring an already significantly demented patient for evaluation and treatment present a quite different problem. Once the diagnosis is established, the family should be educated about the disease and the practicalities of treatment. Depending on the family dynamics, this educational process can take place easily or with great difficulty. The therapist must be alert to the fact that the family will, at least at the beginning, be desperately looking for cures. Support and understanding are necessary. Family members may find participation in one of the growing number of Alzheimer support groups valuable. However, if the primary caregiver is denying the realities of the disease, a support group may provoke anxiety and even increase the level of denial.

Even if the patient lives alone with the caregiver, scheduled family meetings are useful, when possible. At times the meetings may include not only the close relatives such as children or siblings but friends and neighbors as well. During the group meetings, communication difficulties must be clarified. For example, it is not unusual for members of the family to project onto the caregiver their own feelings of depression and anger, frequently accusing the caregiver of aggravating the disease. Family therapy can help by allowing a modulated catharsis of what is often a significant degree of hostility among family members.

When a demented patient is hospitalized or institutionalized, all involved relatives should meet, not only to begin proper support of the patient and family, but also to plan for discharge. The staff of a geriatric psychiatric unit is often helpful in such meetings. An opportunity is also provided to help educate the family about the changing clinical course that will follow and about the anticipated ramifications for patient, family, and significant others.

As Alzheimer's disease progresses, the question of placement in a nursing home or in a setting with more protective care increasingly arises. Depending on the patient's symptoms and the family situation and resources, the need and timing for a transition to a congregate living or nursing home setting will vary. At a certain point, the magnitude of patient dysfunction, limitations of the support system, and/or stress on the family may make the nursing home an inevitable and appropriate choice. This is a situation where families typically experience much ambivalence and guilt, and can benefit enormously from supportive psychotherapy.

BEHAVIORAL INTERVENTIONS

Several techniques have been devised to attempt to train patients with Alzheimer's disease to overcome their deficits. These techniques utilize different forms of intense training, conditioning, or stimulation to help patients utilize their remaining cognitive skills more effectively. The explicit goal of these programs is usually to help the Alzheimer patient learn new skills and behaviors, or relearn lost skills. In some situations, there will be two added benefits from application of these methods. First, they involve the Alzheimer patient more intensely with family and caregivers; when the patient perceives this involvement and support, his or her level of functioning may improve. Second, these programs provide a focus for the family's concern and efforts, and may help them to overcome their feelings of helplessness and guilt as they deal with the progression of Alzheimer's disease. Although these programs may not slow the progession of the dementia, in the proper circumstances they may help to control or reduce certain specific behavior problems that cause excess disability or morbidity. Some of these methods are discussed below.

Reality Orientation

This technique involves intensive attempts by a staff of therapists to orient the Alzheimer patient to his or her environment. It can be a difficult program to institute, requiring the commitment of the entire staff of a nursing home or hospital ward. Such a program uses many methods to vigorously orient the patient to time, place, and situation. Prominent signs and calendars, classes, and intensive one-on-one contact all can be used to communicate this information. As a patient masters the basic data, individualized instruction on more advanced topics can be added. As discussed in the literature, the technique also requires that the staff never listen to delusional talk without trying to correct the patients' misconceptions and attempting to reorient them (Citrin & Dixon, 1977).

A few studies have shown limited improvement on general mental status testing in patients treated with this technique. Unfortunately, there is little evidence that the benefits of the technique extend beyond orientation to social interaction or self-care (Eisdorfer, Cohen & Preston, 1981). There also have been studies suggesting that the sole benefit of reality orientation comes from patient-therapist interaction, not the specific technique used (Brook, Degun & Mether, 1975). This method does appear to increase some patients' sense of well-being, however, and in this respect it may be a valuable tool. The technique may be worth using in situations where family or caregivers need a structured approach to increase their interaction with a patient suffering from Alzheimer's disease.

Conditioning Techniques

Operant conditioning has been used with some success in modifying the behavior of some demented patients. In this approach, a careful behavioral assessment of the patient is undertaken to identify specific behavioral problems. These might include failure to dress, eat, or properly use bathroom facilities, or tendency to engage in socially unacceptable behaviors such as screaming, striking out, or talking about delusions. Once specific behaviors are targeted, a reward strategy is devised that increases the likelihood that the desirable behavior will increase in frequency, thereby replacing an undesirable one.

Such conditioning techniques have been utilized in a number of different situations with elderly patients. There have been several reports of success in increasing socialization, food intake, proper dressing, and exercise among elderly patients in nursing homes (Richards & Thorpe, 1978; Storandt, 1978). Few studies have tried to apply these methods specifically to patients with Alzheimer's disease, but have simply looked at the elderly in general or at those in nursing homes. Where they have been applied specifically to problems common among demented patients (e.g., wandering or urinary incontinence), the results have been mixed, with sometimes only slight improvement noted (Eisdorfer et al., 1981).

At least some patients benefit from these techniques. While very little work has been done to determine the characteristics of these patients, degree of motivation and/or cognitive impairment may be the most important factors. These conditioning methods certainly should be used for particularly troublesome behaviors.

Stimulation and Remotivation Therapy

This group of techniques is designed to combat the sensory deprivation, reduced environmental stimulation, and isolation that can affect a number of older persons in later life, while aggravating the clinical course of those with dementia (Cherkin & Riege, 1983). A few investigators have thus exposed Alzheimer patients to intensive physical and occupational therapy, exercise programs, and other recreational activities. There have been indications that such programs are of slight benefit in improving general memory scores, although there is no evidence that general mental status or ability to perform self-care improves (Eisdorfer et al., 1981).

Remotivation therapy has been used in somewhat less impaired Alzheimer patients in an attempt to increase these patients' awareness of the external environment (Eisdorfer & Stotsky, 1977; Feil, 1967). Regular group therapy sessions are held to discuss current events, literature, or other topics of general interest. This technique, which is designed to increase the confidence, feelings of self-worth, and social interactions of demented patients, has not been demonstrated to be effective in improving cognitive functions (Zarit, 1980).

These techniques can be used by the family in an attempt to interact with the patient and to reinforce his or her remaining cognitive functions. Both methods (activities and discussion) may be appropriate to apply in the home environment and may improve the social situation. Both of these therapies may be most appropriate at early stages of Alzheimer's disease, when patients are more intact and capable of social interactions. Although neither technique appears effective in combating cognitive losses, other psychological benefits (e.g., combating depression, increasing sense of mastery) may be significant and should be considered from a quality-of-life perspective.

Cognitive Training

Some investigators have attempted to train patients with Alzheimer's disease to improve their memory and thinking skills. A variety of specific approaches have been attempted. One technique is imagery training, where the patient uses visual imagery in an attempt to bolster the functioning of failing verbal memory. Other techniques attempt to teach elderly patients new thinking or other memory strategies. These methods, while they have been of some success in the general geriatric population, have not been of help in patients with Alzheimer's disease or other types of dementia. Research in this area nonetheless continues (Zarit, 1980).

Methods Targeted at Specific Behaviors

The family and caregivers of the patient with Alzheimer's disease can frequently develop a limited, practical program to modify, reduce, or eliminate certain behaviors that are dangerous to the Alzheimer patient or a problem for others in the home. The first step toward developing such a program is identification of the particular problems that the patient is having. Some of the more frequent problems are wandering, urinary incontinence, or leaving the stove on or the refrigerator open. Next, a careful assessment can be undertaken to identify the psychological deficits that are causing the problems. For example, is the patient's primary problem a poor memory? If so "memory prostheses" can be used to encourage certain activities or limit others. If the patient has trouble remembering to perform such specific tasks as regular toileting, alarms can be set to go off at certain intervals to remind the patient. If a patient needs to remember to turn off a stove, close the door, or not to leave a room, signs can be put up to stimulate performance of the tasks or to limit activity. Some of these prostheses obviously require that the patient be sufficiently attentive and intact to notice and comprehend the stimulus.

Another major problem for some Alzheimer patients is emotional lability. Some patients can become extremely agitated, violent, or tearful throughout the day. These symptoms, commonly interpreted as depression, may simply represent a difficulty adjusting to the environment. An assessment of the cause may help eliminate the problem. For instance, patients with aphasia may become upset because of their failure to comprehend language. If so, stimuli can be limited, and communication through brief spoken or written phrases can be used. Other patients may become upset because when they are moved to strange surroundings or exposed to new people. For these individuals, keeping them in a constant, structured environment may be helpful (Ware & Carper, 1982).

As Alzheimer's disease progresses, the patient may lose these abilities and more concrete steps must be taken. Doors may have to be locked so that they cannot be opened; knobs may have to be removed from stoves; eventually, the patient may have to be moved to an environment where the dangers for the patient and others can be more completely controlled (see section on chronic institutional settings).

THE USE OF MEDICATION IN DEMENTED PATIENTS

When approaching treatment of the patient with Alzheimer's disease, it is most appropriate to start by considering medications that the patient is already receiving. Drugs are the most frequent cause of delirium and reversible dementia in the elderly, and the Alzheimer patient may be taking several medications that exacerbate his or her cognitive losses (Cummings & Benson, 1983). Most elderly patients take a number of prescription medications. Although they comprise only about 11% of the population, geriatric patients account for more than 25% of all prescribed medications in the United States (Hollister, 1981). More than 40% of the prescription medications commonly used by the elderly can cause significant intellectual impairment or make mild impairment appear more severe (Maletta, 1980), and individuals with multiple medical problems may take several such medications. Classes of drugs most often implicated include tranquilizers, sedatives, antihypertensives, and analgesics.

The problem can be compounded by self-medication. Many elderly patients take over-the-counter preparations to help with sleep, relieve pain, or treat a cold. Many of these medications have strong anticholinergic effects or are highly sedating, and thereby can either cause or contribute to confusion (acute confusional state or delirium).

For many reasons, the elderly are much more susceptible to developing confusion on standard therapeutic doses of many medications. An increase in the ratio of fat to lean body mass, a decline in body water content, a decline in the level of serum proteins binding drugs, slower and less complete drug metabolism, and a slower rate of renal excretion with aging can all contribute to the rapid development of a dementia syndrome by causing higher than usual plasma blood levels of these drugs (Greenblatt, Sellars & Shader, 1982). Demented patients also have increased central nervous system sensitivity to many medications, possibly due to diminished functional brain mass and a concomitant increase in the sensitivity of binding sites for psychotropic drugs. All of these factors can combine to potentiate the effects of even a small dose of a large number of medications. The benzodiazepines, frequently prescribed for sleep and anxiety in the elderly, are often implicated in delirium for a combination of these reasons (Dorsey, 1979), so too are drugs having a high frequency of anticholinergic side effects such as neuroleptics, tricyclic antidepressants, antihistamines, etc.

There is no way to anticipate whether an individual patient will have an adverse reaction to a particular medication. Such reactions are idiosyncratic and unpredictable. In treating the Alzheimer patient, the psychiatrist should therefore simplify medication regimens as much as possible by using the fewest drugs in the lowest effective doses. Since it is frequently difficult to distinguish between effects of an illness and untoward drug effects in the elderly, the physician should always consider the possibility of reducing or discontinuing a given drug, even if just on a trial basis. If the patient has been taking a drug with a potential for fostering dependency (e.g., diazepam), the psychiatrist must be alert for withdrawal symptoms (e.g., severe agitation, sleeplessness) that could be construed as worsening dementia. Another treatment option is to replace one member of a class of medication with another that has a more desirable pharmacokinetic profile. For instance, a physician might choose to replace one sedative (e.g., diphenhydramine) with another that has a shorter half-life and fewer anticholinergic side effects (e.g., temazepam).

Individualizing Drug Treatment

There is a great need, particularly in the patient with Alzheimer's disease, to individualize drug treatment. This need for individualization is due to several factors. First, patients will have differing sensitivities to the therapeutic and toxic effects of medications. For example, some patients will develop confusion or urinary retention while taking thioridazine; others will tolerate this drug well, but will become tremulous and rigid while taking haloperidol. Some elderly patients will have noticeable side effects from all members of a class of drugs. In these cases, the choice of drug may be dictated by which side effects are the least offensive.

Second, patients will have different rates of metabolism for these drugs. For example, one patient might sleep through the night with a short-acting benzodiazepine (e.g., oxazepam), while another requires a longer acting drug (e.g., alprazolam) to avoid early awakening. Information about drug metabolism can usually only be determined empirically, so that it may be necessary to try several different medications in one class.

Third, some patients with Alzheimer's disease will have one or more general medical illnesses that contraindicate certain drugs or change the required dosage. Some patients with severe cardiovascular disease may not be able to tolerate high doses of an antidepressant. Others, however, who are taking coumadin may need higher doses because of increased hepatic metabolism. Medical monitoring of such patients with EKGs, serum drug levels, or other tests may be necessary.

Drug and Somatic Treatment of Behavioral Symptoms

The patient with Alzheimer's disease only rarely suffers from cognitive losses alone. The recognition of memory impairment is frequently followed by feelings of depression and anxiety. As cognitive loss and disorientation progress, the patient may develop sleep disturbance, a major depressive episode, or even psychosis. Such symptoms are very typical of many Alzheimer patients and can cause them to appear much more disabled than they would be from uncomplicated dementia alone. These behavioral symptoms are often responsive to treatment (often to behavioral approaches, at times to a combination of behavioral and pharmacologic interventions)—even in patients with advanced Alzheimer's disease. There have been few controlled trials of the effectiveness of the anxiolytics, antidepressants, and neuroleptics in demented patients (Merriam et al., 1988), but there is a wealth of empirical data to support their efficacy in general (Reisberg, Ferris & Gershon, 1980).

Treatment of Anxiety and Sleep Disturbance. When the patient with Alzheimer's disease complains of anxiety and/or difficulty sleeping, these problems must be carefully evaluated. In its milder forms, anxiety may manifest as complaints of restlessness, agitation, fidgeting, or inability to sit still; in a more severe case, the patient may complain of "wanting to crawl out of my skin." The patient with sleep disturbance may openly complain of the problem, or may simply be found wandering during the night or sleeping during the day.

Although sometimes isolated findings, any of these complaints may also represent the first signs of a major depressive episode. Whether they are isolated findings or symptoms of another major mental illness, the psychiatrist has a range of psychotherapeutic and psychopharmacologic treatment options available.

Medications should not be the immediate, first step in the demented patient with insomnia or anxiety since these drugs can foster dependency and have a number of side effects. Prior to drug treatment, other factors must be considered. Is the patient sleepless or anxious because of difficulties dealing with his or her illness? Is the patient taking medications or drinking caffeinated beverages that might cause insomnia or anxiety? Does the patient have medical problems which, if unrecognized or poorly treated, may manifest with anxiety (e.g., undiagnosed infections such as of the bladder or lungs) or insomnia (e.g., prostatic hypertrophy with urinary frequency)? Has the patient adopted habits which may disrupt normal sleep patterns (e.g., daytime napping)? If the answer to one or more of these questions is yes, psychotherapy, medical management, or counseling may be the most appropriate treatment.

When the physician has determined that medications are necessary, several different classes of drugs can be considered: the minor tranquilizers (e.g., oxazepam), the sedative-hypnotics (e.g., chloral hydrate), or the antihistamines (e.g., hydroxyzine). When these medications are used, it is generally advisable to choose a short-acting agent that has no active metabolites (e.g., oxazepam, lorazepam, alprazolam, or temazepam). Such medications can give a rapid therapeutic effect and are less likely to accumulate in the body causing confusion (Salzman, 1981). Some patients who metabolize these drugs rapidly may suffer rebound anxiety or sleeplessness a few hours after a dose of the medication. A longer acting medication should then be prescribed for these individuals.

Caution must be followed in the use of any of these drugs. Although the goal of treatment frequently is sedation, achievement of this goal may cause other problems. Patients with Alzheimer's disease may become increasingly confused or delirious on even small doses of these sedating medications, especially those with anticholinergic properties (Liston, 1982). This problem can be exacerbated if the medications are administered at night when Alzheimer patients already are most susceptible to confusion.

Sedating drugs, therefore, may lead to a paradoxical increase in agitation that is mistakenly attributed to worsening dementia. This paradox may prompt the physician to increase a medication that is best discontinued. A general rule that is helpful in prescribing these medications, and those discussed below, is to prescribe for the elderly patient one-third to one-half the "standard" dosage for a young adult, and to increase the dosage slowly, taking into account the time necessary to reach serum "steady-state." To calculate steady-state, multiply the half-life in hours times 5, which gives the time necessary to reach serum steady-state at a given dose and frequency of administration (Salzman, Shader & Harmatz, 1975). Patients on these medications should be closely monitored for confusion or worsening agitation.

It may be possible to eliminate anxiety and sleep disturbance completely by following the above-mentioned guidelines. Many patients, however, will not receive complete symptom relief. In some cases, the demented patient will not be able to tolerate sufficiently large doses of these medications for control of symptoms. In other cases, psychological or situational problems must be resolved before anxiety and sleep disturbances can be ameliorated.

Treatment of Severe Agitation or Psychosis. If the patient does not respond to treatment with the drugs mentioned above, if the agitation is severe or associated with psychosis, or if the patient cannot tolerate anxiolytic drugs, one of the neuroleptics may be indicated. Such patients may present with extreme irritability, frequent wandering, screaming, hostility, or even assaultiveness. A frequent problem among Alzheimer patients is "sundowning," or confusion which is exacerbated by the diminished sensory stimulation at night. This problem appears particularly amenable to treatment with the neuroleptics (Ford & Jarvik, 1979), while treatment of sundowning with sedative-hypnotics may actually make the confusion worse. Giving neuroleptics at night can have the added benefit of aiding sleep, although they are not the treatment of choice for simple sedation.

Despite the wide use and reported efficacy of these medications, there is little research on their effectiveness. Barnes and colleagues (1982) found only seven placebo-controlled studies of the effectiveness of these medications in demented patients. In their study, Barnes et al. found only moderate improvement in global behavior in the neuroleptic-treated patients, and only when a few specific behavioral items were scored (anxiety, excitement, emotional lability, and uncooperativeness) was drug superior to placebo. Although there is abundant clinical evidence that neuroleptics are of benefit for Alzheimer patients with delusions and hallucinations, use of the medications in these patients has not been systematically studied. In general, clinical and research results suggest that the neuroleptics should be used only for specific clinical indications.

Thioridazine has been among the neuroleptics most frequently administered to demented patients (Felger, 1966; Reed, 1971). It is among the more sedating of the neuroleptics, and some clinicians report it to be particularly effective in controlling psychosis and agitation (Salzman et al, 1975; Zawadski, Glazer & Lurie, 1978). Thioridazine has the disadvantage, however, of being among the most anticholinergic of the neuroleptics, sometimes causing urinary retention, sedation, and confusion (Barnes et al., 1982; Davis, 1981). It has also been associated with cardiovascular problems, most notably postural hypotension and arrhythmias. These side effects may limit the maximum dosage that can be achieved.

Some of the higher potency neuroleptics (e.g., haloperidol, thiothixene, and fluphenozine) are significantly less anticholinergic and less sedating. Haloperidol has been shown to be equally or more effective than thioridazine in the control of agitation and psychosis among demented patients (Rosen, 1979; Smith, Taylor & Linkous, 1974). Barnes and colleagues (1982) found that loxapine was as effective as thioridazine for control of agitation and psychosis. Unfortunately, these low-dose/high-potency drugs do cause a higher incidence of extrapyramidal side effects (also called EPS, or "drug-induced Parkinson's disease") than the lower potency drugs. The elderly have been reported to be particularly susceptible to extrapyramidal side effects (Fann & Wheless, 1981), although with the low dosages usually required such reactions can often be avoided. In some patients, however, EPS cannot be avoided. Such patients may be at high risk for falling because of their diminished mobility.

The initial dose of any neuroleptic should be small in the elderly. As little as 10 mg of thioridazine or 0.25 mg of haloperidol or 2 mg of trifluoperazine per day may be effective. Such a small dose will actually be therapeutic for some patients. Others will require increases, but the psychiatrist can anticipate that only a moderate total dose will be needed (less than 6 mg of haloperidol, and less than 300 mg of thioridazine) (Spira et al., 1984). A single daily dosage (if tolerated) is frequently sufficient for the control of symptoms, and administration of this dose at bedtime may reduce the complaints of side effects. For the patient with sundowning, the dose may be administered in the early evening before the usual nocturnal confusion develops.

Unfortunately, for many Alzheimer patients, the choice of a neuroleptic is a choice between medications with different unpleasant side effects. Some patients will be better able to tolerate anticholinergic side effects, while for others EPS will be less problematic. The risks and benefits of using the neuroleptics must also be weighed carefully because of the risk of developing tardive dyskinesia. The risk for this disfiguring, potentially irreversible movement disorder increases with age, and is a serious risk in the elderly with even low doses of any neuroleptic (Smith et al., 1978; Task Force on Late Neurologic Effects of Antipsychotic Drugs, 1980). There is no effective treatment.

Although many patients with Alzheimer's disease clearly benefit from neuroleptics, these drugs may be administered too readily to many demented patients. This conclusion was supported by Barton and Hurst (1976), who conducted a double-blind study of chlorpromazine and placebo in 50 demented geriatric patients, who had all received neuroleptics for long periods of time. At the end of the study period, the hospital staff was unable to differentiate the two groups on the basis of symptoms. Barton and Hurst concluded that many elderly demented patients receive major tranquilizers unnecessarily.

The psychiatrist should not hesitate to prescribe adequate doses of the neuroleptics for patients who benefit, since in those cases where the Alzheimer patient must be controlled, chemical restraint is usually preferable to physical restraint. Treatment must be closely monitored, however, to ensure that the benefits are significant and sustained. Some patients may require the drugs only at certain stages of their disease or on an "as needed" basis. For those patients in whom the targeted behaviors are infrequent, chronic adminis-tration of the neuroleptics may not be justified. Other patients may experience no therapeutic effects, and their condition may even worsen with neuroleptics. "Drug holidays" (tapering and then discontinuing a drug and not readministering it unless necessary) may be useful to help document benefits if the psychiatrist is uncertain.

Treatment of Mood Disorders. Serious depression is common in patients with Alzheimer's disease, occurring in anywhere from 15% to 55% of affected individuals (Liston, 1979; Reifler, Larson & Hanley, 1982). It is important to differentiate these depressions, which may require somatic therapy, from sadness and grief, which are frequent reactions among patients with Alzheimer's disease and which are not likely to respond to somatic therapy. This differentiation can be very difficult. Symptoms such as sleep dis-turbance and loss of appetite, weight, and interest—reliable symp-toms of depression in most patients—can be due to either depression or dementia and may therefore be of little help in the differential diagnosis. Furthermore, the Alzheimer patient's diminished level of function or inability to communicate may mask a depressive episode when present. The psychiatrist, therefore, may need to rely more heavily on clinical judgment than on diagnostic criteria in assessing the depressed Alzheimer patient. If the patient has a severe or persistent disturbance in mood, treatment of depression may be appropriate even if the complete picture of a depressive episode is not present. Conversely, an apparent depressive episode may represent only the debilitating effects of Alzheimer's disease.

The antidepressants have been reported to be effective in treating depression among demented patients on the basis of empirical evidence, but there has been little systematic study of their effectiveness (Miller, 1980; Raskind & Storrie, 1980). Cole and colleagues (1983), in their review of the literature, found few studies that specifically addressed the question of antidepressant effectiveness in demented patients, although most studies concluded that the drugs were at least moderately effective. Almost all of these have examined only the tricyclic antidepressants; the monoamine oxidase inhibitors (MAOIs) have hardly been studied in this patient group.

Many of the same cautions that apply to the use of the anxiolytics and neuroleptics apply to the use of the antidepressants as well— including the standard practice approach of considering behavioral or psychotherapeutic approaches first and then combining them with pharmacologic interventions if the latter are indicated. Many of these drugs, particulary the tricyclics, are extremely anticholinergic and may worsen confusion in patients with Alzheimer's disease. The anticholinergic effects of these medications may be especially poorly tolerated by patients with narrow angle glaucoma or prostatic hypertrophy. The sudden increase in intraocular pressure or worsening of urinary retention sometimes caused by these drugs may constitute a medical emergency. Those antidepressants with strong quinidine-like effects (e.g., tricyclics) also may be contraindicated in patients with certain cardiac conduction defects. Patients with A-V block are particularly at risk for the development of complete heart block or heart failure on such medications.

In general, it is advisable to use antidepressants with the fewest anticholinergic side effects (e.g., desipramine, nortriptyline, or trazodone). Trazodone is also reputed to have the benefit of very low cardiotoxicity, but the sedation that it causes may be poorly tolerated by these patients. Most of the antidepressants can be safely administered to most patients with heart disease, although serial electrocardiograms may be necessary to ensure patient safety. For patients with severe cardiovascular disease, inpatient cardiovascular monitoring may be appropriate and ECT can be considered (see below).

There is little information regarding the antidepressant dosage most effective in elderly patients. According to Jarvik and co-workers (1982), older patients are reported to require lower doses of some antidepressants, but there has been no research on dosages required in patients with Alzheimer's disease. The initial dosage for these drugs should be low (10 to 25 mg, or up to 50 mg for trazodone), with the total daily dose likely to fall between 50 and 150 mg

(Salzman and van der Kolk, 1984). Increases should be done carefully, taking into consideration steady-state and related factors.

There are also no data on the time required for antidepressants to be effective in patients with Alzheimer's disease. The psychiatrist should allow at least the same amount of time advised for nondemented patients (3–6 weeks) before concluding that a particular medication is not effective. In addition, for refractory patients or those with significant side effects, the psychiatrist should consider obtaining serum drug levels. Serum drug levels at least can confirm that the patient is taking the medication and that it is being absorbed.

Hypomania or mania also can occur in patients with dementia, and the psychiatrist should follow the same principles that guide treatment in a nondemented patient. If the patient is suffering from a first manic episode, it is important to perform a careful medical evaluation. The new onset of this disorder in old age may represent the first sign of a tumor or other intracranial lesion.

In treating the manic Alzheimer patient, neuroleptics may be used for control of acute symptoms. Lithium carbonate may be effective for long-term control of symptoms. Demented patients may be particularly susceptible to lithium neurotoxicity, however, and may develop confusion, nausea, tremor, and ataxia with low serum levels. Toxicity poses a special problem in these individuals, since it may be difficult to differentiate a toxic confusional state from dementia (Prien & Gershon, 1981). This problem can be magnified in the presence of medical illness such as cardiac or renal disease. Patients who are taking diuretics, who are on salt-restricted diets, or who have diminished creatinine clearance are at greater risk for lithium toxicity. It may be necessary, therefore, to use considerably lower serum levels in such patients; a level as low as 0.3 mEq per liter can be effective in certain patients.

Electroconvulsive Therapy (ECT). Electroconvulsive therapy (ECT) is effective in the treatment of depression in the elderly; it has also been reported as effective in the treatment of depression coexisting with Alzheimer's disease (Snow & Wells, 1981). However, the administration of ECT to Alzheimer patients has not been well studied. ECT causes some reversible memory loss and confusion in most elderly patients, and it is possible that the Alzheimer patient is more susceptible to these side effects. For this reason, when treating the depressed Alzheimer patient, the psychiatrist may want to use ECT only when the patient cannot tolerate medications, when drug treatment along with the other major interventions have failed, or when there is an immediate life-threatening depression.

In any case, the procedure should be carefully discussed with both the patient and family so that they do not become unduly alarmed when confusion or memory impairment develop and mistakenly interpret these side effects as signs of worsening dementia. Evidence from patients with uncomplicated depression indicates that these side effects are reversible, but the question has not been studied in patients with Alzheimer's disease. The psychiatrist may decide that unilateral electrode placement is preferable to bilateral placement in these patients, since the former apparently causes less memory loss. Unilateral placement may also be less effective, however, and extend the total number of treatments required. The preferred method for administering ECT to these patients has not been determined.

Medications for the Improvement of Cognition

Many medications have been tried over the years for the treatment of the cognitive losses of Alzheimer's disease. A few of these have had mild, transient, positive effects on memory and cognition in some patients. Treatment is equivocally helpful to various patients, but current research may lead to more effective treatments. The most promising or researched options for treatment are discussed below.

Vasodilators. This class of drugs has been the most studied over the years. In the 1960s, dementia was believed to be caused by cerebral arteriosclerosis and the consequent diminution of blood flow to the brain. Medications with vasodilatory properties were, therefore, examined in an attempt to increase blood flow to the brain. Subsequently, it has been recognized that the great majority of cases of dementia are due to Alzheimer's disease and that decreases in cerebral blood flow are only secondary to decreases in brain metabolism (Obrist, 1972).

Several of the vasodilators have been described as having some positive effects on cognition that are, however, unrelated to their vasodilatory effects. Foremost among these is a mixture of dihydrogenated ergot alkaloids (dihydroergotamine, or Hydergine). Originally believed to be a vasodilator, then a mild antidepressant, the drug is now thought to act primarily by enhancing nerve cell metabolism since it improves glucose and oxygen utilization in brain tissue (Gaitz, Varner & Overall, 1977; Meier-Ruge et al., 1978). A number of studies have demonstrated that the drug leads to statistically significant improvements on scales measuring such items as alertness, ambulation, mood, and short-term memory (Cook & James, 1981).

Dihydroergotamine is relatively well tolerated, and has been given in doses ranging from 3 to 6 mg. There is no agreement on the optimal dosage nor on how long the drug must be administered before therapeutic effects are apparent (Kugler et al., 1978; Reisberg et al., 1980). The medication appears most likely to benefit mildly impaired patients. Most patients probably derive little benefit from dihydroergotamine, and there are no predictors of which individuals will benefit. Furthermore, some of the reported improvements are of doubtful clinical significance (Hughes, Williams & Currier, 1976). Given the relative safety of this medication, its high cost (Zawadski et al., 1978) is the major obstacle to its routine use.

Other vasodilators have been used as well, but they generally have been found to be ineffective or inferior to dihydroergotamine. One of the most studied is papaverine, a naturally occuring opium alkaloid without morphine-like activity. This drug is a mild vasodilator, but its therapeutic effects have been attributed to dopamine blocking activity (Branconnier & Cole, 1977a). Several controlled studies have demonstrated that papaverine has beneficial effects on cognition and memory and reverses some of the EEG slowing seen in dementia (Branconnier & Cole, 1977b; McQuillian, Lopec & Vibal, 1974). Other studies, however, have found papaverine less effective than dihydroergotamine (Bazo, 1973; Rosen, 1975).

Other vasodilators that have been used in the treatment of dementia include cyclandalate, isoxsuprine, and niacin. There is little support in the literature for the effectiveness of these medications in ameliorating cognitive losses (Neshkes & Jarvik, 1983).

Central Nervous System Stimulants. Several investigators have reported striking abnormalities in the noradrenergic neurotransmitter systems in the brains of patients with Alzheimer's disease (Bondareff et al., 1987; Mann et al., 1980). These findings, along with the lethargy and withdrawal noted in many of these patients, have led to trials of psychostimulants for the treatment of dementia.

The most extensively studied has been pentelenetetrazol. This medication has not been demonstrated effective for the treatment of cognitive losses (Crook, 1979). Other reports concern methylphenidate, magnesium pemoline, denol, gerovital H-3, as well as caffeine. Although there is abundant anecdotal evidence of their beneficial effects, controlled studies have failed to document clinical benefits of these medications in reversing the cognitive losses of dementia (Reisberg et al., 1980). Some of the improvements may be due to antidepressant effects. In a study of gerovital as an antidepressant, however, Olsen, Bank and Jarvik (1978) found that gerovital was not significantly different from placebo in effectiveness. The antidepressant properties of the other stimulants have not been systematically studied.

Neurotransmitters. Researchers have found greatly diminished levels of acetylcholine and activity of the enzyme responsible for its synthesis (choline acetyl transferase, or CAT) in the brains of Alzheimer patients (Davies & Maloney, 1976; McGeer et al., 1984). These deficits have been shown to correlate with the degree of dementia (Perry et al., 1978). The involvement of the cholinergic system has led to trials of acetylcholine precursors and agonists in Alzheimer patients on the theory that enhancement of cholinergic activity may be therapeutic in the same way that enhancement of dopaminergic activity is helpful in Parkinson's disease.

In attempts to increase intracerebral acetylcholine levels, some investigators have utilized dietary loading with the precursors lecithin and choline. Dosages of up to 50 g daily have been given for periods of up to 6 months, but this approach generally has failed to produce significant effects on the memory of demented patients (Brinkman & Gershon, 1983; Thal et al., 1981).

A second approach has been to inhibit acetylcholine degradation with the acetylocholinesterase inhibitor physostigmine.This drug has been of slight benefit to the memory of some demented patients (Mohs & Davis, 1982; Thal & Fuld, 1983), but its short duration of action, narrow therapeutic window, and the requirement for intravenous administration have made its routine use impractical (Terry & Katzman, 1983). An oral form of the drug has recently become available, and one preliminary study indicates that it may improve memory in certain Alzheimer patients without significant toxicity (Mohs et al., 1985).While this improvement was statistically significant, it did not lead to improved function among the patients studied. Still, these results are encouraging and warrant further investigation of orally administered physostigmine. Tetrahydroaminoacridine (THA) is another acetylcholinesterase inhibitor that has had some preliminary positive reports (Summers et al., 1986), though earlier studies found its effect to be little different than that of physostigmine (Kaye et al., 1982). Further studies on THA are in process.

A third approach involves the use of choline agonists such as arecholine. Used systemically, this has produced mild, time-limited improvements at the expense of toxic side effects (Christie et al., 1981). Bethanechol recently was administered through intraventicular injection to four Alzheimer patients and reportedly led to behavioral improvements in three of them without systemic toxicity (Harbaugh et al., 1984). Studies are now underway to determine whether the benefits described in the preliminary report can be reproduced or are of sufficient magnitude to justify either clinical interest or the risks of cranial surgery and infection.

Other Medications. A number of other medications have been tried over the years for treatment of dementia with little or no success. Some of these are discussed briefly below.

Several efforts have been made to manipulate the endogenous neuropeptide systems of the brain in order to influence cognition. The first attempts involved administration of exogenous ACTH or vasopressin; unfortunately, neither drug had significant effect on cognitive functions of demented patients (Durso et al., 1982; Will, Abuzzahab & Zimmerman, 1978). Trials of the endogenous opioid antagonist naloxone have also been conducted. Despite promising initial reports, this treatment has not proved beneficial in the majority of patients (Blass, Riding & Drachman, et al., 1983; Spar, 1984).

Another drug that has been used with mixed results is piracetam. In a few studies, this GABAminergic agonist has been reported to be of slight benefit to various mildly demented patients, although overall it has not been found superior to placebo (McDonald, 1982).

Drug Combinations. A promising new approach to drug treatment of cognitive loss is use of drug combinations. While many of the above drugs have been found to be ineffective individually, there is some evidence that their effectiveness is potentiated by other medications. Physostigmine and lecithin in combination, for example, are noticeably more effective than either alone, though overall changes remain slight, time-limited, and occur in only certain Alzheimer patients (Peters & Levin, 1979). Other combinations now being studied include piracetam and dihydroergotamine, lecithin and physostigmine, and arecholine and physostigmine (Cherkin & Riege, 1983).

TREATMENT SETTINGS AND THE ROLE OF THE PSYCHIATRIST

As the needs of the patient with Alzheimer's disease evolve with the stages of the illness, settings for care may vary—from outpatient treatment to acute medical or psychiatric hospitalization, and finally to chronic institutionalization. Medical, psychiatric and social services often lack coordination and comprehensiveness, leaving patients and families to care that can be insufficient or fragmented. The potential role for the psychiatrist is thus large and challenging. Accordingly, it is important to review the indications for use of a range of outpatient, inpatient, community-based, and institutional settings for care—with attention to the role of the psychiatrist in each.

Outpatient Treatment Settings

Many people with Alzheimer's disease are cared for at home and in the community rather than in institutions. The psychiatrist, therefore, often sees patients and their families in a private office or a clinic, and, at times, in the patient's home. Psychiatric care may include a diagnostic workup, family therapy, individual psychotherapy, psychopharmacologic management, group therapy, and consultation to other care providers. Knowledgeable interventions, including referral to appropriate community services and the provision of respite inpatient care when needed, can maximize the ability of the family to care for the patient.

A number of community services may be available to the patient with Alzheimer's disease living at home, some of which may not involve a psychiatrist. Certain hospitals, clinics, or communities have geriatric outreach teams that visit homes to assess needs for services and to provide crisis intervention and referral; a similar service can be provided by the local Visiting Nurses Association (VNA). Many families will benefit from joining self-help/mutual support groups; the Alzheimer's Disease and Related Disorders Association (ADRDA) has chapters nationwide, in addition to local groups run by hospitals and churches. Groups of senior citizens may also have organized to operate day programs and provide assistance with shopping, cooking, and cleaning. If specific care is needed, physicians may request home nurses, nurses' aides, companions, or rehabilitative therapy to provide medical treatments, medication supervision, bathing, dressing, toileting, the monitoring of vital signs, and exercise.

Special programs may be available. Day care programs (some with psychiatric consultants) can provide social services, activities, group therapy, medication supervision, and meals, while allowing family caregivers part-time respite during workdays. A few communities have centers providing "partial hospitalization" for intensive but less than 24-hour care to adjust medications, monitor behavioral changes, and the like.

Chronic Institutional Settings

Housing that includes services for the elderly can provide a safe environment with peers, recreation, and social services in the building. Often a nurse is available on the premises and transportation is provided. This can be appropriate for patients in earlier stages of Alzheimer's disease or who have a spouse who can provide some but not total assistance.

Board and care facilities (retirement homes) comprise a range of facilities providing room and board with some personal care supervision (e.g. cooking, laundry, dressing).

Nursing homes (skilled nursing facilities and intermediate care facilities) are of major importance in the consideration of treatment settings for Alzheimer's disease patients. It has been estimated that more than half of the elderly in nursing homes have dementia, many of the Alzheimer's type. Skilled nursing facilities provide more intensive care with 24-hour care and treatment supervised by registered nurses. Twenty-four hour care is also provided in intermediate care facilities ("health-related facilities") but with less intensive medical and nursing care.

The psychiatrist may serve as a consultant caregiver of patients in nursing homes, providing diagnostic workup, medication management, and supportive family therapy. Educational guidance for staff (e.g., on the use of orientation aids such as calendars, clocks, radios, family photos, and on the management of wandering or agitated patients) may be needed as well. Nursing homes vary in their ability to tolerate disruptive behavior, from screaming to incontinence, on the part of Alzheimer patients. Generally, very demented patients who do not need acute hospitalization have difficulty finding appropriate settings.

The decision to place a patient at home or in a nursing home can be critical. The needs, resources, and desires of each patient and family are quite individual. The possibility of long-term placement in a nursing home may arise when the patient has no primary caregiver, or when the severity of the illness precipitates a crisis as by incontinence or by behavior that is self-endangering, assaultive, or psychotic. It may be necessary to transfer the patient to a nursing home if the crisis cannot be adequately addressed through outpatient interventions. Such interventions include medication adjustments, partial hospitalization, respite care to assist temporarily overwhelmed caregivers, other supplemental services, or acute hospitalization. The appropriate nursing home should be able to provide the intensity of care needed by the individual, should be experienced in caring for Alzheimer's disease patients, and should be accessible to the family.

Psychotherapeutic Approaches within Psychiatric Hospitals

The indications for psychiatric hospitalization of the Alzheimer's patient vary according to the stage of the disease. In relatively early stages when suicidal depression may be a factor, the patient clearly requires hospitalization. Conversely, it is not uncommon to see depressed elderly admitted to the hospital and in the ensuing workup be diagnosed with Alzheimer's disease. If the presentation is sufficiently ambiguous, diagnosis may be best accomplished in the psychiatric unit.

Anorexia and agitation frequently necessitate hospitalization later in the disease. If a therapeutic alliance has previously been established, psychotherapeutic techniques can be useful in resolving the problems in the hospital; it is much more difficult when the psychiatrist first sees such a patient in the hospital. Finally it is often useful for a family that is no longer capable of handling wandering, incontinence, and episodic agitation to have the patient hospitalized and perhaps medicated while the family is seen in psychiatric consultation to help them adjust to the institutionalization of the patient. Such an approach enhances the likelihood of a smoother disposition, whether a return to the community or ongoing institutionalization.

The choice of psychiatric unit depends to a large extent on the geographical location. In urban medical centers, there has been a significant increase in the number of geriatric psychiatry units. Such units have the advantage of especially skilled staff and good medical backup. In small communities, the general psychiatry unit is most often used. If the demented Alzheimer patient is the only elderly patient hospitalized on a medical or surgical service, it may be necessary to provide one-to-one care. The family at times can assist in this capacity.

If there is at least a small number of elderly, the inclusion of Alzheimer's disease patients into intensive therapeutic milieu group meetings as described can be useful in the integration of these patients into the therapeutic community (Nathan, 1973). Frequently these Alzheimer patients enter into somewhat successful reciprocal relationships with other patients in the hospital community.

A mixture of all ages, from adolescence to senescence, can be a good demography for therapeutic work. Sharp age and functioning differences (adolescents and older demented patients), however, may not work as well since the patients may split into two distinct communities. Although such problems are less important on geropsychiatric units, there is frequently a split between the demented and the functional patients. In community meetings, patients can be invited to discuss their behavior problems such as nighttime wandering, forgetting the location of the bathroom, and urinary incontinence. If these difficulties are handled in a nonthreatening way, there can sometimes be remarkable support and advice from the group.

Because the structure of the psychiatric unit can vary so widely, it may be best to outline the milieu features that would be optimal for demented patients. These features include:

1. Not isolating the demented patient (via restraints or keeping them in the most remote part of the unit).

2. Adequate staff to contain disruptive behavior.
3. Brief structured programs to avoid overstimulation or confusion.
4. Significant individual direction (may even be provided by other patients).
5. A multidisciplinary team approach to facilitate the assessments and treatment.
6. Staff and a unit milieu which is understanding of the behaviors.
7. Safe environment (on a unit with agitated or violent young schizophrenics, elderly patients are often afraid or actually abused); also, an environment that can accommodate though contain wandering.

All activities are directed by the treatment team which may consist of the psychiatrist, psychiatric nurse, psychiatric social worker, psychologist, family therapist, and at times creative arts therapists. Psychiatric nurses play a critical role in the treatment of these patients, not only for the psychological but also the physical care of the patient. The nurse's close contact with patients has proved valuable in reestablishing meaningful communications with seemingly hopelessly demented patients. Such contact should be a model for all caregivers. When close professional attention is combined with noncognitive treatment, such as music, movement, and art therapy, patients seem less anxious and somewhat better cognitively.

Psychiatric hospitalization of Alzheimer patients is usually acute. Under such circumstances nursing home placement is generally not indicated. This should be clarified to the family as soon as possible during the hospitalization, especially since the nursing home issue can be charged for both patient and family. Accordingly, significant attention must be paid to preparing patient and family for the eventual discharge. Counseling is often extremely useful to the family in providing support and direction in their handling of the patient. The hospitalization of entire families has been tried experimentally with reported success (Eisdorfer & Stotsky, 1977).

Most facilities, however, must be content with regular weekly (or less often) family visits. Posthospital treatment planning is important because, for Alzheimer's disease patients, this is frequently a lifetime commitment.

The Demented Patient in the General Hospital — The Role of the Liaison Psychiatrist

Although demented patients requiring hospitalization should perhaps ideally be treated in psychiatric hospitals, they often find their way into general hospitals. It is not uncommon for an acute medical problem to bring the Alzheimer's disease patient to a general hospital. Reports on geropsychiatric consultation offer some data on the presence of demented elderly in these settings. There is, however, considerable variation in the reports. One study (Ruskin, 1985) of 67 patients, age 60 or older, described dementia in 19% of the subjects and delirium in an additional 18%. Another study of 329 geriatric consultations (Nathan, 1985), which represented 22% of all consultations over the age of 65 for a 2-year period, showed a 39.5% rate of dementia and a 7% rate of delirium among the patients. This study also found that the overall admission rate to the hospital of patients 65 and over was 36%. Distinct from these findings that followed psychiatric consultation, the hospital's overall discharge data revealed that only 2.7% of the elderly patients had diagnoses of any degree of dementia. The discrepancy from the consultation data, and from the higher frequency of dementing disorders in the elderly reported by formal epidemiological studies of the population as a whole, may be explained by a lack of general medical awareness of mild dementia, including its potentially reversible forms. Frequently, early signs are dismissed as "just old age." In addition, a hopeless attitude concerning dementia still too often appears in primary care settings, almost as if there is nothing that can be done to help. In general, in this setting the percentage of patients reported to have a primary or secondary diagnosis of dementia at discharge varies across studies, further reflecting the varied preparedness of staff in dealing with such patients.

There are several reasons for admitting an Alzheimer's disease patient to a general hospital. These include the need for a differential diagnostic evaluation and a functional assessment. Dementia patients are also admitted for general medical problems that cause excess disability or become less well managed because of the patient's cognitive impairment. Regardless of the clinical scenario, the role of the psychiatrist can be critical, whether in clarifying diagnosis, helping to establish the level of functioning capability, or in assisting with the management of dementia with other clinical disorders.

There are also issues of how to help staff better manage these patients while they are hospitalized. On a medical floor, some of the methods of dealing with these patients include reviewing behavioral management techniques such as simple orienting exercises, family consultation, medication where indicated (usually for agitation) along with contact and recommendations for the referring physician; the latter should focus not only on hospitalization issues but also on posthospitalization planning.

Another important issue is that of ongoing education for nonpsychiatric personnel. Such training can boost both staff skills and morale. Behavioral management approaches and techniques for better orienting demented patients to time and place can make a big difference for both patient care and staff satisfaction in being able to make a difference. In many centers there is a high turnover of nursing personnel associated with low levels of inservice training, highlighting the need to teach these techniques on a regular basis for the ever-changing staff.

The nature of the hospital setting is compounded by such demanding clinical problems as sensory overload or understimulation, immobilization, consciousness-altering medications, pain, delirium, and dementia. This already difficult clinical situation is sometimes made even more difficult by the problem of differentiating delirium from dementia (Lipowski, 1983). The treatment of the delirious demented patient must begin with the elimination of the possible causes of the delirium and requires a close relationship with medical colleagues.

The medical staff in hospitals, perhaps because they are unaware of the capacities of demented elderly, often unknowingly reject such patients. Since one aspect of liaison work is education, it is hoped that the presence of an interested psychiatrist dealing with a demented patient, seeing that patient regularly, and discussing the progress of the patient with the medical housestaff and attending physician would at least attenuate the tendency toward rejection. A more fundamental solution could be effected during the education of students and residents. Many students, notwithstanding their high level of education, are unaware of how much patients can vary in terms of their orientation, memory and ability to relate in a warm and friendly manner. The introduction on a liaison consultation rotation of medical students and psychiatric residents to the diagnostic and treatment potential of demented patients frequently results in a significant change in attitude toward such patients.

A medical hospitalization may be the first indication to members of the family that a spouse or parent has been diagnosed as having Alzheimer's disease. The attending physician should be encouraged to discuss the diagnosis and prognosis with the family. A psychiatric consultant at the discussion can set a tone of realistic expectation that might otherwise be missing.

The extended family can be called in to family meetings and family resources mobilized to support the patient and the primary caregiver. It is important to make clear to the family as well as to medical professionals associated with the patient and family that, although Alzheimer's disease is not curable, it is treatable; clinical interventions can alleviate symptomatology and patient suffering at different points along the course of the disorder, while helping to reduce family burden and stress.

REFERENCES

Altschuler, K., Barad, M., & Goldfarb, A. (1963). A survey of dreams in the aged. II. Noninstitutionalized subjects. *Archives of General Psychiatry, 8,* 33–37.

Barnes, R., Veith, R., Okimoto, J., et al. (1982). Efficacy of antipsychotic medications in behaviorally disturbed dementia patients. *American Journal of Psychiatry, 139,* 1170–1174.

Barton, R., & Hurst, L. (1976). Unnecessary use of tranquilizers in elderly patients. *British Journal of Psychiatry, 112,* 989–990.

Bazo, A.J. (1973) An ergot alkaloid preparation (hydergine) versus papaverine in treating common complaints of the aged: Double blind study. *Journal of the American Geriatric Society, 21,* 63–71.

Bellak, L., Hurvich, M., & Gedimen, H. (1973). *Ego functions in schizophrenics, neurotics and normals.* New York: John Wiley.

Blass, J.P., Riding, M.J., Drachman, D., et al. (1983) Opiate antagonists in patients with Alzheimer's disease. *N. Engl. J. Med., 309,* 354–355.

Bondareff, W. Mountjoy, C.Q., Roth, M., Rossor, M.N., Iversen, L.L., Reynolds, G.P., & Hauser, D.L. (1987). Neronal degeneration in locus ceruleus and cortical correlates of Alzheimer's disease. *Alzheimer Disease and Associated Disorders, 1,* 256–262.

Branconnier, R., & Cole, J.O. (1977a). Effects of chronic papaverine administration on mild senile organic brain syndrome. *Journal of the American Geriatric Society, 25,* 458–462.

Branconnier, R., & Cole, J.O. (1977b). Senile dementia and drug therapy. In K. Nandy & I. Sherwin (Eds.), *Advances in Behavioral Biology: The Aging Brain and Senile Dementia.* (Vol. 23). New York: Plenum.

Brenner, C. (1982). *The mind in conflict.* New York: International Universities Press.

Brinkman, S.D., & Gershon, S. (1983). Measurement of cholinergic drug effects on memory in Alzheimer's disease. *Neurobiology of Aging, 4,* 139–145.

Brody, E. (1985). The Kent lecture. *The Gerontologist, 25* (1), 19–29.

Brook, P., Degun, G., & Mether, M. (1975). Reality orientation, a therapy for psychogeriatric patients: A controlled study. *British Journal of Psychiatry, 127,* 42–45.

Brosin, H.W. (1952). Chapter contributions of psychoanalysis to the study of organic cerebral disorders. In F. Alexander & H. Ross (Eds.), *Dynamic psychiatry.* Chicago: University of Chicago Press.

Butler, R.N. (1960). *Intensive psychotherapy for the hospitalized aged. Geriatrics, 15,* 644.

Cherkin, A., & Riege, W.H. (1983). Multimodal approach to pharmacotherapy of senile amnesias. In J. Cervos-Navarro & H.I. Sarkander (Eds.), *Brain aging: Neuropathology and neuropharmacology.* New York: Raven Press.

Christie, J.E., Shering, A., Ferguson, J., et al. (1981). Physostigmine and arecholine: Effects of intravenous infusions in Alzheimer presenile dementia. *British Journal of Psychiatry, 138,* 46–50.

Citrin, R.S., & Dixon, D.N. (1977). Reality orientation. A milieu therapy used in an institution for the aged. *The Gerontologist, 17,* 39–43.

Cohen, D., & Eisdorfer, C. (1986). *The loss of self.* New York: Norton.

Cole, J.O., Branconnier, R., Salomon, M., et al. (1983). Tricyclic use in the cognitively impaired elderly. *Journal of Clinical Psychiatry, 44,* 14–19.

Cook, P., & James, I. (1981). Cerebral vasodilators. *New England Journal of Medicine, 305,* 1508–1513.

Crook, T. (1979). Central-nervous-system stimulants: Appraisal of use in geropsychiatric patients. *Journal of the American Geriatric Society, 27,* 476–491.

Cummings, J.L., & Benson, D.F. (1983). *Dementia: A clinical approach.* Boston: Butterworths.

Davies, P., & Maloney, A.J.R. (1976). Selective loss of central cholinergic neurons in Alzheimer's disease. *Lancet II*, 1403

Davis, J.M. (1981). Antipsychotic drugs. In T. Crook & G. Cohen (Eds.), *Physicians' handbook on psychotherapeutic drug use in the aged.* New Canaan, CT: Mark Powley.

Dorsey, F.G. (1979). Overview of aging and risk of susceptibility to pharmacologic iatrogenic problems in the elderly. In A.J. Levenson (Ed.), *Neuropsychiatric side effects of drugs in the elderly.* New York: Raven Press.

Durso, R., Fedio, P. Brouwers, P., et al. (1982). Lysine vasopressin in Alzheimer disease. *Neurology, 32,* 674–677.

Eisdorfer, C., Cohen, D., & Preston, C. (1981). Behavioral and psychological therapies for the older patient with cognitive impairment. In N.E. Miller & G.D. Cohen (Eds.), *Clinical aspects of Alzheimer desease and senile dementia. Aging, (Vol. 15).* New York: Raven Press.

Eisdorfer, C., & Stotsky, B.A. (1977). Intervention, treatment, and rehabilitation of psychiatric disorders. In J.E. Birren & K.W. Schaie (Eds.), *Handbook of the psychology of aging* (1st ed., pp. 724–748). New York: Raven Press.

Engel, G. (1962). *Psychological development in health and disease.* Philadelphia: Saunders.

Fann, W.E., & Wheless, J.C. (1981). Treatment and amelioration of psychopathologic affective states in the dementias of late life. In N.E. Miller & G.D. Cohen (Eds.), *Clinical aspects of Alzheimer's disease and senile dementia. Aging (Vol. 15).* New York: Raven Press.

Feil, N.W. (1967). Group therapy in a home for the aged. *Gerontologist, 7,* 139–141.

Felger, H.L. (1966). Thioridazine in the geriatric patient. *Diseases of the Nervous System, 27,* 537–538.

Ford, C.V., & Jarvik, J.F. (1979). The treatment of dementia and depression in the elderly. *Advances in Primary Care, 18,* 1–6.

Gaitz, C.M., Varner, R.M., & Overall, J.E. (1977). Pharmacotherapy for organic brain syndrome in late life. *Archives of General Psychiatry, 34,* 839–845.

Gallagher, D. (1987). Caregivers of chronically ill elders. In G.L. Maddox (Ed.), *The encyclopedia of aging.* New York: Springer.

Goldfarb, A.I., & Turner, H. (1953). Psychotherapy of aged persons. II. Utilization and effectiveness of brief therapy. *American Journal of Psychiatry, 109,* 916.

Goldstein, A. (1939). *The organism.* New York: American Book.

Greenblatt, D.J., Sellars, E.M. & Shader, R.I. (1982). Drug disposition in old age. *New England Journal of Medicine 306,* 1081–1088.

Grotjahn, J.M. (1940). Psychoanalytic investigation of a seventy-one year old man with senile dementia. *Psychoanalytic Quarterly, 9,* 80–97.

Group for the Advancement of Psychiatry. (1971). *The aged and community mental health: A guide to program development* (Vol. 8, series 81). New York: GAP.

Harbaugh, R.E., Roberts, D.W., Coombs, D.W., et al. (1984). Preliminary report: Intracranial cholinergic drug infusion in patients with Alzheimer's disease. *Neurosurgery, 15,* 514–518.

Hartmann, H. (1961). *Ego psychology and the problem of adaptation.* (D. Rappaport Transl.). New York: International Universities Press.

Hauser, S. (1978). Ego development and interpersonal style in adolescence. *Journal of Youth and Adolescence, 7,* 333-352.

Hollister, L.E. (1981). General principles of psychotherapeutic drug use in the aged. In T. Crook & G. Cohen (Eds.), *Physicians handbook on psychotherapeutic drug use in the aged.* New Canaan, CT: Mark Powley.

Hollos, S., & Ferenczi, S. (1925). *Psychoanalysis and the psychic disorder of general paresis.* New York: Nervous and Mental Disease.

Huges, J.R., Williams, J.G., & Currier, R.D. (1976). An ergot alkaloid preparation (hydergine) in the treatment of dementia: Critical review of the clinical literature. *Journal of the American Geriatric Society, 24,* 490-497.

Jarvik, L.F., Mintz, J., Steuer, J., et al. (1982). Treating geriatric depression: A 26-week interim analysis. *Journal of the American Geriatric Society, 30,* 713-717.

Kaye, W.H., Sitaram, N., Weingartner, H., Ebert, M.H., Smallberg, S., & Gillin, J.C. (1982). Modest facilitation of memory in dementia with combined lecithin and anticholinesterase treatment. *Biological Psychiatry, 2,* 19-26.

Kugler, J., Oswald, W.D., Herzfeld, U., et al. (1978). Long-term treatment of the symptoms of senile cerebral insufficiency: A prospective study of hydergine. *Deutsche Medizinische Wochenschrift Stuttgart, 103,* 456-462.

Lewin, B. (1950). *The psychoanalysis of elation.* New York: Norton.

Lewis, J.M., & Johansen, K.H. (1982). Resistances to psychotherapy with the elderly. *American Journal of Psychotherapy, 36*(4), 497-504.

Lipowski, Z.J. (1983). Transient cognitive disorders (delirium, acute confusional states) in the elderly. *American Journal of Psychiatry, 140,* 1426-1436.

Liston, E.H. (1979). Clinical findings in presenile dementia: A report of 50 cases. *Journal of Nervous and Mental Diseases, 167,* 337-342.

Liston, E.H. (1982). Delirium in the aged. In L.F. Jarvik & G.W. Small (Eds.), *Psychiatric Clinics of North America* (Vol. 5). Philadelphia: W.B. Saunders.

Mace, N.L., & Rabins, P.V. (1981). *The 36-hour day.* Baltimore: Johns Hopkins University Press.

Maletta, G. (1980). Use of psychotropic drugs in the older patient. In G. Maletta & F. Pirozzolo (Eds.), *The aging nervous system.* New York: Praeger.

Mann, D.M.A., Lincoln, J., Yates, P.O., et al. (1980). Changes in the monoamine containing neurons of the human central nervous system in senile dementia. *British Journal of Psychiatry, 136,* 533-541.

McDonald, R.J. (1982). Drug treatment of senile dementia. In D. Sheatley (Ed.), *Pharmacology of old age.* London: Oxford.

McGeer, P.L., McGeer, E.G., Suzuki, J., et al. (1984). Aging, Alzheimer's disease, and the cholinergic system of the basal forebrain. *Neurology, 34,* 939-944.

McQuillan, I.M., Lopec, C.A., & Vibal, J.R. (1974). Evaluation of EEG and clinical changes associated with Pavabid therapy in chronic brain syndrome. *Current Therory and Research 16,* 49-58.

Meier-Ruge, W., Emmenegger, H., Enz, A., et al. (1978). Pharmacologic aspects of dihydrogenated ergot alkaloids in experimental brain research. *Pharmacology Suppl. 1, 16,* 45-62.

Merriam, A.E., Aronson, M.K., Gaston, P., Wey, S., & Katz, I. (1988). The psychiatric symptoms of Alzheimer's disease. *JAGS, 36,* 1-6.

Miller, N.E. (1980). The measurement of mood in senile brain disease: Examiner ratings and self-reports. In J.O. Cole & J.E. Barrett (Eds.), *Psychopathology in the aged.* New York: Raven Press.

Mohs, R.C., & Davis, K.L. (1982). A signal detectability analysis of the effect of physostigmine on memory in patients with Alzheimer's disease. *Neurobiology of Aging, 3,* 105–110.

Mohs, R.C., Davis, B.H., Johns, C.A., Mathe, A.A., Greenwald, B.S., Horvouth, T.B., & Davis, K.L. (1985). Oral physostigmine treatment of patients with Alzheimer's disease. *American Journal of Psychiatry, 142,* 28–33.

Nathan, R.J. (1973). The psychiatric treatment of the geriatric patient. *American Journal of Psychiatry, 130,* 711–714.

Nathan, R.J. (1985). The geriatric patient in the consultation liaison service. A paper presented to the Pennsylvania Psychiatry Society, Harrisburg, Pennsylvania.

Nathan, R.J. Rose-Itkoff, C., & Lord, G. (1981). Dreams, first memories, and brain atrophy in the elderly. *Hillside Journal of Clinical Psychiatry, 3*(2), 139–148.

Neshkes, R.E., & Jarvik, L.F. (1983). Pharmacologic approach to the treatment of senile dementia. *Psychiatric Annals, 13,* 14–30.

Obrist, W.D. (1972). Cerbral physiology of the aged. Influence of circulatory disorders. In C.M. Gaitz (Ed.), *Aging and the brain.* New York: Plenum.

Olsen, E.J., Bank, L., & Jarvik, L.F. (1978). Gerovital H-3: A clinical trial as an antidepressant. *Journal of Gerontology, 33,* 514–520.

Ory, M.G., Williams, T.F., Emr, M., Lebowitz, B., Rabins, P., Salloway, J., Sluss-Radbaugh, T., Wolff, E., & Zarit, S. (1985). Families, informal supports and Alzheimer's disease: Current research and future agendas. *Research on Aging, 7,* 623–644.

Peters, B.H., & Levin, H.S. (1979). Effects of physostigmine and lecithin on memory in Alzheimer disease. *Annals of Neurology 6,* 219–221.

Perry, E.K., Tomlinson, B.E., Blessed, G., et al. (1978). Correlations of cholinergic abnormalities with senile plaques and mental test scores in senile dementia. *British Medical Journal, 2,* 1457–1459.

Prien, R.F., & Gershon, S. (1981). Lithium. In T. Crook & G. Cohen (Eds.), *Physicians' handbook on psychotherapeutic drug use in the aged.* New Canaan, CT: Mark Powley.

Rabins, P.V., Mace, N.L., & Lucas, M.J. (1982). The impact of dementia on the family. *Journal of the American Medical Association, 248*(3), 333–335.

Raskind, M., & Storrie, M.C. (1980). The organic mental disorders. In E.W. Busse & D.G. Blazer (Eds.), *Handbook of geriatric psychiatry.* New York: Van Nostrand Reinhold.

Reed, M. (1971). Psychopharmacology in the geriatric patient. *Rocky Mt. Medical Journal, 68,* 44–48.

Reifler, B.V., Larson, E., & Hanley, R. (1982). Coexistence of cognitive impairment and depression in geriatric outpatients. *American Journal of Psychiatry, 139,* 623–626.

Reifler, B.V., & Wu, S. (1982). Managing families of the demented elderly. *Journal of Family Practice, 14*(6), 1051–1056.

Reisberg, B., Ferris, S.H., & Gershon, S. (1980). Pharmacotherapy of senile dementia. In J.O. Cole & J.E. Barrett (Eds.), *Psychopathology in the aged*. New York: Raven Press.

Richards, W.S. & Thorpe, G.L., (1978). Behavioral approaches to the problems of later life. In M. Storandt, I.C. Siegler & M.F. Elies (Eds.). *The clinical psychology of aging*. New York: Plenum.

Rosen, H.J. (1975). Mental decline in the elderly. Pharmacotherapy-ergot alkaloids versus papaverine. *Journal of the American Geriatric Society 23*, 169–174.

Rosen, H.J. (1979). Double-blind comparison of haloperidol and thioridazine in geriatric outpatients. *Journal of Clinical Psychiatry, 40*, 17–20.

Ruskin, P.E. (1985). Geropsychiatric consultation in a university hospital: A report on 67 referrals. *American Journal of Psychiatry, 42*, 333–336.

Salzman, C. (1981). Antianxiety agents. In T. Crook & G. Cohen (Eds.), *Physicians' handbook on psychotherapeutic drug use in the aged*. New Canaan, CT: Mark Powley.

Salzman, C., Shader, R.I., & Harmatz, J.S. (1975). Response of the elderly to psychotropic drugs: Predictable or idiosyncratic? In S. Gershon & A. Raskin (Eds.), *Aging* (Vol. 2). New York: Raven Press.

Salzman, C., & van der Kolk, B. (1984). Treatment of depression. In C. Salzman (Ed.), *Clinical geriatric psychopharamacology*. New York: McGraw-Hill.

Schilder, P. (1953). *Medical psychology*. (D. Rappaport Trans.). New York: International Universities Press.

Smith, G.R., Taylor, C.W., & Linkous, P. (1974). Haloperidol versus thioridazine for the treatment of psychogeriatric patients: A double-blind clinical trial. *Psychosomatics, 15*, 134–138.

Smith, J.M., Oswald, W.T., Kucharski, L.T., et al. (1978). Tardive dyskinesia: Age and sex differences in hospitalized schizophrenics. *Psychopharmacology, 58*, 207–211.

Snow, S.S., & Wells, C.E. (1981). Case studies in neuropsychiatry: Diagnosis and treatment of coexisting dementia and depression. *Journal of Clinical Psychiatry, 42*, 439–441.

Spar, J.E. (1984). Psychopharmacology of Alzheimer's disease. *Psychiatric Annals, 14*, 186–189.

Spira, N., Dysken, M.W., Lazarus, L.W., et al. (1984). Treatment of agitation and psychosis. In C. Salzman (Ed.), *Clinical geriatric psychopharmacology*. New York: McGraw-Hill.

Storandt, M. (1978). Other approaches to therapy. In M. Storandt, I.C. Siegler & M.F. Elies (Eds.), *The clinical psychology of aging*. New York: Plenum.

Summers, W.K., Majovski, L.V., Marsh, G.M., Tachiki, K., & Kling, A. (1986). Oral tetrahydroaminoacridine in longterm treatment of senile dementia, Alzheimer type. *New England Journal of Medicine, 315*, 1241–1245.

Task Force on Late Neurological Effects of Antipsychotic Drugs. (1980). Tardive dyskinesia: Summary of a task force report of the American Psychiatric Association. *American Journal of Psychiatry, 137*, 1163–1172.

Terry, R.D., & Katzman, R. (1983). Senile dementia of the Alzheimer type. *Annals of Neurology, 14*, 497–506.

Teusink, J.P., & Mahler, S. (1984). Helping families cope with Alzheimer's disease. *Hospital and Community Psychiatry, 35*(2), 152–156.

Thal, L.J., & Fuld, P.A. (1983). Memory enhancement with oral physostigmine in Alzheimer's disease. *New England Journal of Medicine, 308,* 720.

Thal, L.J., Rosen, W., Sharpless, N.S., et al. (1981). Choline chloride fails to improve cognition in Alzheimer's disease. *Neurobiology of Aging, 2,* 205–208.

Verwoerdt, A. (1981). Individual psychotherapy in senile dementia. Clinical aspects of Alzheimer's disease and senile dementia. In N. Miller & G. Cohen (Eds.), *Aging* (Vol. 15). New York: Raven Press.

von Bertalanffy, L. (1974). General system theory and psychiatry. In S. Arieti (Ed.) *American handbook of psychiatry* (2nd ed., Vol. I, pp. 1095–1117). New York: Basic Books.

Ware, L.A., & Carper, M. (1982). Living with Alzheimer disease patients: Family stresses and coping mechanisms. *Psychotherapy Theory, Research and Practice, 19,* 472–481.

Will, J.C., Abuzzahab, F.S., & Zimmerman, R.L. (1978). The effects of ACTH4-10 versus placebo in the memory of symptomatic geriatric volunteers. *Psychopharmacology Bulletin, 14,* 25–27.

Zarit, S.H. (1980). *Aging and mental disorders: Psychological approaches to assessment and treatment.* New York: Free Press.

Zawadski, R.T., Glazer, G.B., & Lurie, E. (1978). Psychotropic drug use among institutionalized and noninstitutionalized Medicaid aged in California. *Journal of Gerontology, 33,* 824–834.

5

CASE EXAMPLES

INTRODUCTION

The ten case examples presented illustrate further the range of clinical issues and opportunities for psychiatric intervention in treating patients and their families with Alzheimer's disease. The capacity of psychiatric treatment to alleviate symptoms, reduce suffering, and maximize functioning for this disorder will thus become more tangible. Similarly, the role of the diverse therapeutic interventions—psychotherapy, behavioral approaches, pharmacotherapy, family therapy, etc.—a psychiatrist can offer in working with these patients will be clearer. Treatment in different settings— home, hospital, nursing home, etc.—will be illustrated.

In these case examples, the terms Alzheimer's disease and primary degenerative dementia will be used interchangeably in response to DSM-III-R (APA, 1987) changes; the abbreviation AD will also be used for Alzheimer's disease. Each example will begin with a brief delineation of key clinical issues that will be addressed such as diagnosis, psychotherapy, pharmacotherapy, and treatment in the nursing home. Each example will then be followed by a brief discussion highlighting some of the major points covered. The case examples will vary in length—some providing a snapshot of an important clinical issue or treatment opportunity, others providing considerably more detail to allow a more in-depth appreciation of process or clinical course.

CASE EXAMPLE 1

Key Clinical Issues

Differentiating depression from dementia in Alzheimer's disease
The role of depression as an "excess disability" factor in Alzheimer's
    disease (290.21, DSM-III-R)
Treatment of excess disability in Alzheimer's disease in the community

The Case

A 75-year-old, brilliant chemist, Professor JB, was evaluated because
of significant trouble he was having with memory and concentration,
to the extent that he no longer could balance his checkbook and
no longer took an interest in reading. JB described difficulty
noticeable only to him a year earlier, when he began to be less
facile with complicated equations. To others he still looked quite
sharp, but not to himself. This problem was a terrible blow to JB's
self-esteem, and he began to experience trouble sleeping, loss of
appetite and weight, and further difficulty concentrating. A thorough differential diagnostic workup ruled out many causes of
dementia-like symptoms that can mimic senile dementia and left
the clinician with the diagnosis of Alzheimer's disease. But the
impression was that depression was also present.

Treatment for the depression was instituted, combining individual psychotherapy once a week and an antidepressant medication
(desipramine, 25 mg three times a day). JB's appetite returned, the
weight loss stopped, concentration improved, and he started reading again, although trouble with the checkbook continued. The
therapeutic work helped JB come to terms with his underlying
disorder, Alzheimer's disease. Residual skills were maximized during that stage in the course of his illness, and quality of life during
that interval was enhanced.

Discussion

This case example dramatically illustrates the remarkable phenomenon of a patient experiencing temporary improvement in functioning while suffering from an underlying progressive illness, and the impact of lifting the excess disability. Depression compounded the dementia, aggravating the degree of cognitive impairment and overall dysfunction, accounting for the excess disability. Following the intervention for the depression, fully another 3 years passed before Professor JB again reached the level of cognitive impairment he had when first seen. Treatment gave him 3 better years at a critical juncture in the course of his life.

CASE EXAMPLE 2

Key Clinical Issues

Delusions as an excess disability factor in Alzheimer's disease (290.20, DSM-III-R), and the response to treatment
Treatment of the Alzheimer patient in the home and in the community
Access to and the therapeutic alliance with the reluctant patient
The role of the home visit

The Case

TM, a 76-year-old woman with Alzheimer's disease, who had lost her husband three years earlier, was having increasing difficulty managing her two bedroom condominium by herself. A working daughter and an older sister who lived in the vicinity provided her emotional support and helped with some of her household responsibilities. However, her increasing incapacity, together with the limits in her daughter's time and her sister's strength, made it necessary for the family to seek home help for her. An effort was made to engage the services of a homemaker. TM resisted this idea, saying that she valued her independence and was sure that some stranger would only interfere in her affairs. She finally relented, but the homemaker was allowed to come for only a week, at which point TM told her not to come back. She was defensive about her actions, explaining that the homemaker was planning to steal her belongings. Efforts to get her to accept a new homemaker proved futile, and the family wondered whether she would be able to continue living alone under these circumstances. At the same time, TM was very resistant to the idea of moving.

Consultation was sought, and TM consented to be examined in her apartment. What emerged during the evaluation was that in addition to a mild-to-moderate degree of memory impairment and difficulty in following through with various chores, TM also revealed covert paranoid thinking that became apparent only on careful probing. She had subtle but significant concerns about a conspiracy going on among unknown parties, aimed at taking over her holdings. The delusions were not challenged directly, which would likely have only provoked the patient at that point and caused her to lose confidence in the therapist. The inner tension that she felt about them was real and considerable, and was accordingly acknowledged. This became the basis of a therapeutic alliance that permitted her to accept the idea of trying some medication that could help her cope better with the stress of her situation. Trifluoperazine, 2 mg three times a day (later reduced to 2 mg at bedtime), was prescribed in conjunction with follow-up supportive psychotherapeutic visits. The delusions subsided, and TM allowed the idea of homemaker assistance to be brought up again. This time she was able to tolerate a stranger coming into her home, and the arrangement worked out. TM died 4 years later, from a heart attack at home. At the time her memory and intellectual impairment had progressed only to a stage of moderate cognitive decline (see chapter on Clinicopathologic Correlations). Had TM not been able to tolerate a homemaker, her cognitive deficits would have been too great to permit the degree of independent living she was able to maintain.

Discussion

This case illustrates the degree to which delusions can compound coping capacity in Alzheimer's disease, showing what improvement can follow if these delusions can be lifted or lightened. Like depression, delusions too can cause excess disability in AD; similarly this form of excess disability also responds to treatment. Different durations of the illness in different individuals can lead to different outcomes. Hence, when the clinical course is long one might die *with* the disease (from other causes) at a less advanced stage, rather than *from* it (as many have suggested) at an advanced stage. In this case, treatment gave the patient better years—with less symptomatology and a higher level of functioning—than would otherwise have been the situation in the course of her illness.

Also apparent in this case is the potential role of the home visit in dealing with the reluctant geriatric patient, reducing problems of access and fostering the establishment of a therapeutic alliance.

CASE EXAMPLE 3

Key Clinical Issues

Diagnostic dilemma
Alzheimer's disease with delirium (290.30, DSM-III-R), depression, and delusions in the same patient
Overall treatment strategies with particular attention to pharmacologic management of depression and delusions in an inpatient setting
Treatment response with lifting of excess disability
Family system and social support issues
Disposition posthospitalization

The First Meeting

MP was a 73-year-old woman who lived with her son in a large house in a deteriorating neighborhood. For 5 years, the crime rate in her neighborhood had increased as the socioeconomic status declined. Within the past year, several of her neighbors and friends had moved away. Her son enrolled at a local college and thus was around the house much less. She had generally been in good health except for deteriorating vision from her cataracts.

For at least 2 years, the friends who still had contact with MP noticed that she was becoming increasingly forgetful and confused. She complained that she would go to the grocery store and forget why she was there. Sometimes she would have to make several trips in one day just to get all the items that she needed. Her son reported that she would call him at least once a week because she had gotten lost while driving; he would then go and help her return home. The neighbors complained that the condition of MP's house was deteriorating, and that garbage was piling up in back. When they complained to MP, she would accuse them of putting the garbage there.

The patient's son noted that she had become increasingly delusional and reclusive over the past 6 months. He had taken her to see her internist, but complained that the doctor had been of little help. Finally, the son brought her to the geropsychiatry outpatient clinic where MP was evaluated and admitted to the hospital.

MP came to the ward with her son. The patient was extremely agitated and said that she was convinced that she was at a prison, not a hospital. She began to cry uncontrollably, screaming that she knew she would be executed. She willingly took medication, however, and was given haloperidol 2 mg orally. She was then taken to her room, and the history was obtained from her son.

The son reported that for more than 6 months prior to admission, MP had been telling him that there were "dope pushers" in the basement of their house making PCP in the furnace. She claimed that these men put her to sleep at night by passing ether through the ventilation ducts so that she would be "out of the way" when they made PCP. MP had told her son that she knew when they were making drugs by the peculiar way that her neighbor would sometimes hang her laundry on the clothesline. In the month before admission, the son reported that his mother's delusions had become more bizarre. She claimed that the dope pushers were shining laser beams into her windows at night, causing the curlers in her hair to heat up.

The son finally convinced his mother to see her internist several weeks before her admission. The internist had evaluated MP briefly and prescribed a combination of chlordiazepoxide and amitriptyline for her in an unknown dosage. The son reported that his mother had worsened on this medication. She became very confused and wandered aimlessly around the house. She claimed to see parts of bodies lying on the furniture. The son had decided that MP had to see a psychiatrist, and she offered little resistance in her very confused state. Despite her protests, she had even agreed to sign for a voluntary admission.

The patient's son was 27 years old; he had continued to live at home because of uncertainty about "what I wanted to do with my life." His mother has supported him financially and did not mind his sharing their rather large house. He believed that his mother had been excessively demanding of him over the prior year, however, and felt that she had been "holding him back" from going out on his own. He seemed irritated when discussing this situation.

MP's son reported that his mother had always been in good health except for her cataracts. She was taking no medications except for the psychotropic. He noted that she had been sleeping much less in the few weeks before admission, but attributed this to her being "worked up over those crazy ideas." He was unaware of any change in her weight or appetite.

At that point the nurse reported that the patient had calmed down enough to be interviewed. Examination revealed MP to be disoriented to place and time. She was poorly attentive and uncooperative with formal mental status testing. She had marked loosening of her associations, jumping from topic to topic unrelated to questioning. She perseverated on the theme of the drug dealers, whom she believed even then were trying to kill her.

Approach to the Diagnosis

MP appeared to have an acute worsening of her mental status in the few weeks prior to admission, marked by confusion as well as auditory and visual hallucinations. This deterioration coincided with initiation of her medication. Given the patient's mental status, a diagnosis of delirium was made.

The patient's history indicated that she had suffered from another major mental illness prior to the onset of the delirium. The present illness was marked by auditory and visual hallucinations as well as paranoid ideation and ideas of reference. These psychotic symptoms occurred in the presence of a history of mild depressive symptoms and increasing cognitive losses. Accordingly, the differential diagnosis included paranoid disorder, major depressive episode with mood-incongruent psychotic features, and dementia.

MP's delirium made it difficult to diagnose her underlying condition. The history was only slightly helpful in sorting through the differential diagnoses. MP suffered from significant life stresses, social isolation, and sensory loss (e.g., cataracts) prior to the onset of her illness. This constellation of factors tended to predispose her to the development of both psychosis and depression. A history of cognitive loss, however, made dementia another possibility.

The treatment team concluded that it was necessary to let the delirium clear before an accurate diagnostic impression could be obtained. The plan was to let the patient detoxify and to treat her agitation as necessary with neuroleptics. When the patient's mental status permitted, she would be interviewed in greater depth. Psychological testing would also be performed to assess the degree of her cognitive losses. In addition, the patient would undergo a thorough general medical evaluation looking for other causes for delirium.

Treatment

The patient was treated with oral haloperidol in doses ranging from 2 to 7 mg for the first three days of her hospitalization. During this time she remained extremely confused and delusional, although somewhat less agitated. She claimed to smell gases that the dope pushers had put into her room to poison her and claimed to see dead bodies in the corners of the room. She frequently wandered around the ward aimlessly, asking for directions. At one point, she approached her physician with an empty patient gown in her arms saying, "Look here, I have the body of my son."

Baseline laboratory studies were obtained. All serum chemistries were within normal limits.

After three days in the hospital, the patient's mental status began to improve. She became oriented to place, and on occasion, to time. She became more attentive, her wandering decreased, and both short- and long-term memory improved. She no longer smelled poison gases or saw dead bodies, but she continued to believe that there were drug dealers who wanted to kill her. There was no longer gross disorganization of her thought or loosening of associations.

With the improvement in her mental status, the patient could be engaged in regular exploratory interviews. During these interviews, MP was found to have a clearly depressed mood and affect. She was able to discuss her feelings of sadness at the loss of her friends, and she was frequently tearful. She seemed particulary saddened by the increasing loss of contact with her son, but noted that it was "his time to leave." MP seemed very agitated while discussing these issues. She would constantly wring her hands, and sometimes got up and paced. Closer questioning of MP revealed that her appetite had decreased notably during the 6 months before admission and that she had lost 15 pounds. She also reported that she had been sleeping poorly.

After another several days, psychological testing was performed. The results showed that the patient had a moderately impaired ability to attend and concentrate. She had mild-to-moderate global cognitive impairment with a score of 22 on the Mini-Mental State Exam (see chapter on diagnosis). Her paranoid delusions were well-circumscribed, and her thinking was logical. Her MMPI showed marked depression with feelings of worthlessness. She endorsed items stating that she felt she was a burden on others.

MP was diagnosed as having a major depressive episode with mood-incongruent psychotic delusions, and possible underlying dementia. Treatment with desipramine was instituted at a dose of 50 mg at bedtime. Supportive psychotherapy was started using brief but frequent meetings with the patient that focused on orienting her to reality and her situation.

Clinical Course

The patient improved steadily following the initiation of desipramine. After 1 week, the dosage had been increased to 150 mg. MP tolerated the medication well. After 2 weeks on the medication, her mood and affect were much brighter and she began to socialize with the other patients. When asked about her delusions she either denied having them or stated, "The dope pushers just don't bother me the way they used to." She continued to demonstrate moderate cognitive impairment. She would sometimes get disoriented on the ward, and frequently misplaced her possessions. While engaged in ward activities, she would occasionally forget what she was doing and required frequent orientation to time.

At that point, MP was seen in regular problem-oriented psychotherapy sessions. The therapy initially focused on the patient's depression over the losses of friends, family, and her cognitive abilities. She had been saddened by the loss of many of her friends and frightened by the loss of her vision. MP had felt that she could cope with these problems because she had her son's help and support. She stated that about a year before admission, however, he seemed less interested in her and became irritated at her request for help. When he told her that he was starting college, she became very frightened that he would move out soon. MP also realized that she could not think or remember as clearly as she once had and was convinced that she would die if he left.

The therapist pointed out to her that her son's growing independence was inevitable, and the patient herself stated that she did not want to "hold him back." MP was fearful of going to a nursing home, however, because she was certain that she would soon die there. The therapist investigated other possibilities with both the patient and her son. MP's finances were limited, however, and she could not afford a live-in companion. Because the patient's disability was only moderate in degree, the possibility of a board-and-care home was discussed. She was reassured that she would be able to maintain much of her independence at that kind of facility, and she responded positively to the suggestion.

It was crucial for MP to have her son's support during that time if her transition to the board-and-care home were to be successful. In a series of therapy sessions, the social worker helped the son realize that while he needed his own independence, his mother's dependence was an understandable reaction to her increasing isolation and deteriorating physical and mental health. Both the patient and her son responded to this approach, and the son agreed to help MP find a suitable board-and-care home.

After several visits to board-and-care homes, MP found a facility that she liked. Her son seemed supportive of her and committed to making the transition as smooth as possible. The patient was discharged after a 4-week hospitalization. The discharge diagnosis was major depressive episode, resolved, and Alzheimer's disease, based on the clinical picture, natural history, and other disorders being ruled out. MP was followed for 6 months through the outpatient clinic and remained free of psychotic symptoms, although she continued to have moderate cognitive impairment.

Discussion

With some Alzheimer patients it may not be clear whether the manifestation of depression represents a clinical subtype of Alzheimer's disease or a second disorder coexisting with the dementia; in either instance, the depression may cause excess disability and may respond to treatment. This case also illustrates how major symptoms in AD can shift at different times in the same patient. Any of several treatment options may alleviate the symptoms.

CASE EXAMPLE 4

Key Clinical Issues

The clinical course of Alzheimer's disease with attention to the
   transition from one's home to the nursing home
The use of environmental manipulation and memory aids in
   managing the memory and behavioral problems of AD
AD with psychosis and associated behavioral problems in the
   nursing home setting
Neuroleptic management of AD with delusions

The Case

DL was a 76-year-old woman who emigrated to the US from Poland
after World War II. She lived for many years with her daughter and
son-in-law in their two-bedroom apartment. She had not worked
since coming to this country, but had been active in some senior
citizen community activities such as weekly card games and concerts.
She had also helped with cleaning and cooking at home.

DL had never been friendly with people outside the home. She
would frequently state that the neighbors did not like her, for many
reasons. Among them were that she was a foreigner, she was Jewish,
and she was smarter than they were. DL had always been suspicious
of people who came to the apartment to visit, saying that she was
not sure why they were there.

Approximately 5 years earlier, her daughter had begun to notice
that DL was becoming more forgetful. After the patient had cleaned
the apartment, many objects were misplaced and sometimes could
not be found for days. Dinners that DL cooked were overseasoned
or burned because she could not remember what ingredients she
had added or how long the food had been cooking. The family
took DL to the geropsychiatry outpatient clinic for an evaluation.
After a thorough workup the diagnosis of Alzheimer's disease was
made. The daughter and son-in-law said that they had expected
this news, and that they were resolved to keep DL at home with
them no matter what happened.

The daughter realized that some changes would have to be made in the household routine if her mother were to continue living at home. She tried to relieve her mother of her household responsibilities but DL balked at this, saying she was not becoming "old and useless." Rather than continuing to fight with her mother about this issue, she observed her mother for a few days to determine what tasks her mother might still be able to perform well. These turned out to be vacuuming the carpets and washing the windows and floors. The daughter told her mother that these were the tasks that she needed special help with. DL then gladly concentrated her efforts on these. Since DL was no longer meticulous about her cleaning, the daughter had a maid come in once a week to thoroughly clean the apartment while her mother was at the senior center.

Soon, DL began to have trouble finding her way around the neighborhood, and was getting lost on her way to the senior center. At first, her son-in-law paid a young neighborhood boy to come and escort DL to and from the center. They never told her that the boy was employed to do this, and DL assumed that he did it because he "had no grandmother of his own." The family instructed DL to stay at home apart from these trips to the senior center, because "we need your help here." After another 5 months, however, DL started trying to leave the apartment regularly on her own, and would always get lost.

The daughter and son-in-law then went through a series of steps to try to keep DL safe at home. They explained to her the need to stay at home, and placed a sign on the door reminding her not to leave. They also took turns calling her every couple of hours to talk for a few minutes.

This plan worked for a few months. Soon, however, DL became less interested in her previous activities. She stopped her cleaning, and would sit around the apartment for hours on end. The only household activity that seemed to interest her was cooking. She no longer wanted to go to the senior center, saying that they "didn't like her," and she became increasingly suspicious of the boy who came to take her there. Her daughter hired a series of companions to come and spend time with her mother during the day. DL was extremely suspicious of them all, however, saying that they were only there to steal from her. She was so abusive to them that none stayed more than 2 weeks.

At this point, her daughter and son-in-law placed DL in a nursing home. After an initial period of a few weeks when she screamed at her daughter about trying to "get rid of me," DL adjusted to the facility surprisingly well. She seemed to enjoy having people around her all the time, even though she said that "none of them are as good as me" and "they only want to steal from me." DL guarded her possessions closely and talked to few people, but seemed calm for the first year in the home.

At the end of this year, she began to tell her daughter about men who came into her room at night with knives and threatened to kill her. These complaints were intermittent and were made without much affect. They seemed to diminish when a large nightlight was installed in her room. After 4 months, however, the hallucinations became much more bothersome to DL. She would sometimes scream at night and wander down the hall, waking people up and asking for help. Once she found an unlocked door, and wandered out "looking for the police." She was found sleeping on a bench the next morning.

At this point, her family brought her back to the geropsychiatry outpatient clinic for an evaluation. They could find no reversible cause for her psychotic symptoms, and she was started on haloperidol 0.5 mg at bedtime. This effected good control of her psychotic symptoms. She complained only occasionally about the nighttime intruders, and even then their presence seemed not to bother her. The dosage was increased once every 4–8 months over the next 2 years because of worsening agitation.

After 2 years in the home, DL assaulted one of the nurses with a table knife. She claimed that she had been watching this "peasant" for the past few months and that the woman was plotting to poison her. At this point, DL's haloperidol dose was up to 3 mg. As it was increased further, she became very stiff and her movements were quite slowed. She had difficulty in getting out of bed. Anticholinergic agents were added to her regimen, but these increased her confusion. The haloperidol was then changed to perphenazine 5 mg at bedtime. DL tolerated this medication much better. It controlled her symptoms well, and the staff reported her to be easier to take care of.

Discussion

Excess disability in AD can be treated both in nursing homes and in the community. Perhaps had the family brought DL in earlier for outpatient treatment, she might have been able to tolerate the "companion" and thereby remain at home longer (as in Case 2, TM, whose delusions interfered with her ability to accept help). This case illustrates some of the many conceivable coping strategies, for example, the family's employment of the boy, the use of signs, and the regular phone calls to help DL structure her day. Psychiatric consultation for developing behavioral and environmental strategies to address problem behaviors in the home as well as the nursing home can be invaluable.

CASE EXAMPLE 5

Key Clinical Issues

Diagnostic dilemma, particularly in the early stage of Alzheimer's disease (Is it dementia or depression? Is it dementia with depression?)
The natural history of Alzheimer's disease
Family system problems

The Case

BB was a 76-year old married woman who lived with her husband in a high-rise apartment building. She was seen initially by the medical staff at the insistence of her daughter for an assessment of memory loss and anxiety of 3 years duration. The onset was insidious, and BB refused to acknowledge that any of her family's concerns were justified. Her son-in-law was a physician who insisted that the symptoms must be manifestations of depression since BB had a 30-year history of recurrent depressions. However, the precipitants and characteristics of prior depressive episodes were always more clear-cut, and responses to pharmacologic interventions for depression were always dramatic. The patient had not responded to antidepressant medication during this episode, suggesting a diagnosis other than depression.

For 2 years, BB was reportedly belligerent when it was pointed out that she had not completed a task or was kept from wandering. She was still able to perform most routine household tasks such as cleaning and shopping and cooking, but was having increasing difficulties with judgment. Despite her daughter's reports of BB's long-standing marital difficulties, which seemed to be worsening as the couple aged, both BB and her husband refused to acknowledge them. There was also a history of alcohol misuse by the patient, which had reportedly stopped 5 years earlier.

BB showed no neurological abnormalities or major general medical diagnoses during a complete medical evaluation. A CT Scan of the brain showed mild cortical atrophy, and EEG showed diffuse slowing which was consistent with a degenerative dementia.

BB was referred to psychiatry services for consultation and psychological testing. WAIS-R, Wechsler Memory Scale, Aphasia Screening Test, TAT, and Rorschach were administered over three test sessions. The patient was able to travel independently to and from the hospital for testing, but seemed very disorganized in test situations. She was cooperative with cognitive tests, but was very guarded on personality tests. She scored in the low-average range on WAIS scores without significant subtest variability. Her aphasia screening was within normal limits, as were writing and copying geometric designs. Projective tests showed nonresponses such as "I don't know" or "I can't think of it." Affect was absent from her responses, and stories had a vague and repetitive quality. She was not readily engaged in the initial interviews, and responded only to direct questions, offering no spontaneous verbalizations.

BB had worked briefly before her marriage as a typist, but stopped after marrying to raise her two children. She had few hobbies or interests and relied heavily on her husband for decisions. BB's family labeled her a dependent personality.

BB was one of 14 children, abandoned by her father before the age of ten. Her marriage of over 50 years had always been strained because of her husband's lack of acceptance of her dependent needs. There were frequent discussions of divorce or separation throughout the marriage, and her husband had known extramarital affairs. This seeming recapitulation of her childhood family situation had not been adequately worked through in her past psychiatric treatments. Additional family tension was present with BB's children, who felt that their parents had been unable to provide adequate emotional support, and felt bitter and angry with them.

When first seen in the psychiatric hospital, BB was diagnosed as having primary degenerative dementia of the Alzheimer's type with depressive features. BB's family showed marked denial. For BB's children, this denial seemed to be related to a growing realization that their childhood wishes could never be realized. For BB's husband, he seemed to be overwhelmed by the caregiving demands and lacked knowledge about the disease.

The treatment plan consisted of three major elements: 1) Enroll BB in a structured daycare center program and provide supportive weekly psychotherapy. 2) Help BB's daughter deal with her depression and guilt regarding her sense of helplessness and her need to mourn unfulfilled wishes about how she wished her relation to her mother could be. Help BB's husband confront his denial and obtain a better understanding of his wife's cognitive deficits and needs. 3) Avoid antidepressants due to the labile nature of BB's moods and to the past failure of such medications. Prescribe haloperidol as needed at times of extreme belligerence.

Course

After 18 months of relative adjustment, there was an acute change in BB's behavior. She refused to go to daycare, became quite paranoid, rigid, and argumentative, and insisted on wearing her best clothes and mink coat eveywhere. Her husband instructed her not to wear her coat, and the patient complied by throwing her coat away. She avoided her husband's criticisms by locking herself in the elevator. This prompted a brief hospitalization.

With the abrupt change in the patient's behavior, it was necessary to reassess the possibility of an acute medical problem or an acute organic brain syndrome, reevaluate her medication regimen, and begin intensive work with the family. General medical causes were ruled out. The history, which was obtained from several sources, suggested that BB had experienced an assault to her self-esteem at the daycare center, and was responding defensively against this. At the time of rehospitalization, her son-in-law again insisted that a pseudodementia was being overlooked. BB's husband became disengaged again, and her daughter became increasingly uncertain and depressed. Addressing these issues was a primary goal of hospital treatment.

BB's functional capacities were retested, diagnostic tests were repeated, and her medications adjusted. Despite confirmation of a deterioration in global functioning without a major depression, the family remained unconvinced. When BB refused to return to the daycare center, home assistance was provided.

Three months after discharge, BB's son-in-law arranged for an out-of-state assessment by other "experts." When the original diagnosis was confirmed, the family felt further psychiatric care was not needed, and the patient was lost to follow-up.

Discussion

Treatment plans for Alzheimer's disease patients may need to be shelved temporarily when external stressors precipitate crises. The patient may then need short-term hospitalization for relief.

Unless the family can work through their reactions to the patient's illness, their reaction patterns may recur. In BB's case, the family, especially her physician son-in-law, resisted and criticized each diagnosis and treatment. When there was no improvement in BB's condition, he continued to blame the psychiatrist for a misdiagnosis. Such reactions are common and should themselves be issues to be resolved in counseling.

Even the diagnosis of organic brain syndrome need not engender hopelessness and assumptions that treatment can accomplish nothing. Premature withdrawal from treatment, as was apparently true for BB, may rob the patient of an opportunity to ameliorate some of the symptoms.

CASE EXAMPLE 6

Key Clinical Issues

Deceptive (atypical) early manifestations of Alzheimer's disease
The natural history of the disorder and changing treatment needs that accompany it
Family system dynamics

The Case

BC was a 67-year-old married woman. After an initial diagnosis of Alzheimer's dementia when she was 64, her husband sought a second opinion. A more comprehensive evaluation was then carried out by a second primary care physician, who sought neurological consultation. No focal neurological features were noted, and the patient's physical examination, EKG, and blood and urine chemistries were all within normal limits. A CT Scan showed no atrophy or evidence of other brain disease, and an EEG was read as normal. A RISA Scan, LP, ANA, and a Dexamethasone Suppression Test were performed, and also determined to be normal. This second workup revealed no other brain disorder or general medical condition, the main findings being from the patient's history, which revealed a past episode of depression and a question of paranoia. Given the possibility of a pseudodementia, pharmacologic intervention was initiated with psychotropic medication. Respective 2-month trials on maprotiline, thiothixene, chlorazepate, alprazolam, diazepam, phenelzine, chlordiazepoxide, and methyl-phenidate, were tried; no response was noted.

Psychiatric consultation was then sought. The patient's major complaints focused on having no ambition and showing progressive social anxiety and withdrawal for several years. She had apparently been well until the age of 60, when she was forced to retire from an assembly job due to factory layoffs. Her husband noted that prior to the layoff, the patient had a 3-year history of persecutory fears about co-workers and neighbors, complaining that she felt they were talking behind her back and trying to humiliate her. She and her husband, who had been married over 40 years, had never had significant outside friendships and had no children.

Further evaluation found BC to manifest word-finding difficulties and a verbal aphasia that interfered with fluency as well as recent memory impairment. At times, she made errors of omission or refused to answer when pressed for factual information. Her predominant affect was anxiety and fearfulness of exposing deficits. She was extremely fearful of being separated from her husband and insisted that he answer her questions for her. She was fearful of being alone and did not travel anywhere without accompaniment, but had no functional incapacities in activities of daily living. More prolonged periods of fearfulness were also portrayed as being accompanied by feeling "quite down."

BC had one prior depressive episode requiring hospitalization shortly after she married; it had responded to ECT. Her father had apparently suffered a "nervous breakdown" in his mid-40s. BC's husband insisted that his wife spoke fluently when she was alone with him and showed no evidence of the impairments that the doctors had reported. He verbally chastised her "for making him look like a fool in front of the doctors." He perceived no pressures on himself and could only be engaged by being seen in conjunction with his wife (who insisted on his being present with her).

A trial on desipramine was initiated in combination with monthly supportive sessions which reviewed the patient's activities and specific problems in relationships. The impression was that the earlier medication trials may have suffered from improper dosage and duration of antidepressant usage on the one hand to the failure to combine drug treatment with supportive individual and family therapy. BC's husband reported this intervention to be helpful, with some improvement in the patient's overall mood, outlook, and general coping skills.

Over the next 2 years, the patient became increasingly aphasic to the point that speech was unintelligible. She no longer followed verbal commands, and developed agraphia, alexia, and apraxias (e.g., in using kitchen utensils). Her manifest anxiety decreased, though she still resisted being separated from her husband. She no longer required antidepressant medication, and became quite compliant. As her disorder progressed, BC showed no increase in anxiety nor any development of delusions. Her requirement for assistance with activities of daily living (ADL) continued slowly to rise. A follow-up EEG after 2 years showed marked diffuse slow wave activity.

At this point, her husband began to look for miracle cures and said, "Though no one believes me, she talks at times as normally as anyone." He stated that he still believed that something could make her well—either science or God. He sought anti-Alzheimer drugs from Europe and Mexico that were not available in the US, but always asked for advice on safety before purchasing any. In this way, he could be advised against the possibility of victimization.

BC's husband would seek no direct counseling or relief for himself. He insisted that he did not feel burdened by his wife, and that there were no substantive changes in his lifestyle due to her illness, since they typically took no vacations and did little outside the house. He would offer no information about himself unless he felt it was presenting information about his wife (e.g., how they met, the activities they did with his family, their "adoption" of their nephews and nieces as godchildren, their disappointment in not having children, etc.). Though he did not want individual sessions, at the point that his wife could no longer communicate and seemed unable to comprehend any speech, he spent "her" entire session discussing his caregiving. When it was determined that his wife could not benefit directly by counseling sessions, he broke into tears to state he did not need help, but he did not want her to be dropped since the doctor she was seeing was her favorite.

Continued supportive sessions were provided for him through the context of treatment for his wife. He was encouraged to keep his wife from becoming isolated, since isolation could further aggravate her condition. This allowed him to accept the idea of her attending a daycare center. With the burden of constant care being alleviated by this arrangement, he was able to maintain some of his business relationships on a part-time basis.

Discussion

Although memory loss is the most common clue suggesting Alzheimer's disease, patients occasionally complain initially of other symptoms. For example, BC's first complaints were behavioral disturbances and speech impairment.

After several years, the patient's recent memory became impaired, accompanied by social withdrawal. As her aphasia worsened and she could not deal with daily tasks, her earlier depression and tendencies toward suspiciousness seemed to lessen. Perhaps a decrease in self-awareness reduced her need for defensive reactions to maintain her self-esteem.

When family members are adversely affected by the burdens of caregiving for an AD patient and by feelings of guilt, treating the family becomes critical and can be quite challenging. As in BC's case, a spouse may deny the illness or the effect of the illness on the family. When the family is centripetally oriented with little outside social engagement, their problems can be compounded. They may turn, as BC's husband did, to a futile search for miracle cures to make the patient well again.

CASE EXAMPLE 7

Key Clinical Issues

Alzheimer's disease with delirium
The clinical course of AD and how an excess disability can affect it
The course of treatment in the community
Symptomatic family member responses to a loved one with AD

Major emotional conflict over nursing home placement of an AD
patient on the part of the patient's spouse

The Case

CF was a 77-year-old married man without children. He was a
retired engineer living in a city apartment with his wife. CF had
been treated for Alzheimer's disease in the outpatient psychiatric
clinic of a university medical center.

Approximately 5 years earlier, the patient's sister-in-law noticed
that CF spoke almost exclusively of events in the past. On a visit to
her home, CF forgot to telephone them from the train station, got
into a car with a stranger, and then could not identify their house.
He began to forget appointments and phone messages and would
lose his way home from doing errands. After 2 years of such
impaired memory, he was seen by a neurologist, who diagnosed
Alzheimer's disease based on a neurological exam and a workup
including a CT Scan. CF's wife cared for her husband at home,
but he gradually became more difficult to manage. A consulting
psychiatrist prescribed a bedtime dose of diazepam.

Several weeks later, Mrs. CF brought CF to the psychiatric emergency room. Having become increasingly disoriented and agitated,
he had tried to leave the house through the window. He no longer
recognized his wife and struck her once. She was afraid she could
no longer care for him at home. On mental status exam, CF was
disoriented in all three spheres, recalled 0/3 objects after one
minute, and was giggling and inappropriate with looseness of
associations, tangential thinking, and auditory and visual hallucinations. Physical exam and laboratory tests were otherwise normal.
He was admitted to a private psychiatric hosptial, where he was
stabilized on chlorpromazine in small doses (50 mg P.O. twice daily)
and started on ergoloid mesylates (1 mg P.O. three times daily). On
discharge some weeks later, he went home and was seen for follow-up
at the medical center psychopharmacology clinic. He was calm and
pleasant on this regimen, still disoriented with poor memory, but
sleeping well and able to be cared for by his wife.

After that, Mr. and Mrs. CF were seen every 2 months at the clinic by a psychiatric resident, who monitored CF's mental status, blood pressure and medication, and provided advice and support to his wife. At that time, the patient knew his name and street address (but not city or apartment number), his birth date (but not age) and his wife's nickname (occasionally he thought she was his mother). He had a friendly childlike demeanor, but had trouble communicating effectively, answering questions with meaningless numbers or statistics. A gradual reduction of his medication came under consideration.

Mrs. CF was an anxious, self-sacrificing, and devoted caregiver whose life centered around her husband's many needs and making financial ends meet. According to Mrs. CF, her own childhood was sad and in her present situation her only living relative was a sister, who she felt was critical of her decision to care for her husband at home. She had only a few friends and had turned away from outside interests. She came regularly to appointments and plunged into a discussion of her requests and concerns. She reviewed locating a sympathetic internist and geriatric dentist, preparing nutritious but soft foods, techniques for dealing with incontinence, her conflicted feelings about applying for home care and/or Medicaid, how best to preserve her husband's dignity and past values, and how to have a vacation. Friends living in a warm climate had the CF's for two brief vacations; they understood the severity of Mr. CF's illness and Mrs. CF enjoyed the change. At home, a nun who visited was a source of support and invited Mrs. CF to telephone her any time, day or night.

The most painful topic for Mrs. CF was placing her husband in a nursing home. She was proud that she had kept him at home and cared for under her high standards. She cried wrenchingly at the thought that, in a nursing home, he might want someone at night, summon them, and no one would hear him. (Typically he would clap his hands or snap his fingers while "bunked" into his bed with rolled sheets so as not to fall out, and Mrs. CF, just a few feet away, would awaken.) She had an awareness that his placement represented his death to her, and she felt that his death would be the loss of all meaning in her life.

Discussion

CF waited for 2 years after the onset of his first dementia symptoms before visiting a physician. Perhaps, as often occurs in older people, his impaired memory was dismissed as "natural." Diazepam, the first medication prescribed, can precipitate a delirium in elderly patients. In this case, the addition of a sedating neuroleptic appeared to have helped the patient by lessening the psychotic symptoms and agitation.

The phenomenon of excess disability in AD is again illustrated, where concomitant symptoms of psychosis or delirium make the patient do worse than with uncomplicated dementia. When the excess disability is treated, clinical improvement can occur, and with it may come an increased capacity to remain in the community longer.

In this case, the mesh of the spouse's temperament and needs with the patient's needs allowed this patient to be cared for at home despite incontinence, edentulousness, and severe memory deficits. In cases like this, the spouse can also be assisted by support group help (to gain emotional support from families in similar situations and to lessen any sense of isolation), respite care services (for periodic reprieves from the degree of responsibility and burden), access to partial hospitalization services (should serious symptom flare-ups occur, such as episodes of delirium or difficult-to-manage psychotic episodes), consultations to help with painful decisions and transitions concerning nursing home placement and, eventually, the death of patient.

CASE EXAMPLE 8

Key Clinical Issues

Psychiatric crisis in the spouse of the Alzheimer patient
The "spend down" crisis in the financing of care in Alzheimer's disease

The Case

WW was a 73-year-old European-born man, a married but childless retired jeweler living alone in an apartment in a run-down area of a major city. He was brought to the psychiatric emergency room of a medical center near his home by a worried resident physician from the ophthalmology clinic, who had seen WW for a complaint of blurry vision. WW had expressed to the resident a wish to give rat poison first to his wife and then to himself.

WW had never before met with a psychiatrist and was deeply humiliated by the evaluation. He directed frequent devaluing comments to the psychiatric resident and attending physician. With graying hair and a proud bearing, dressed in plain but neat winter clothes, WW refused to take off his woolen jacket and denied that his rat poison statement had been more than a joke. After some time, however, he gradually revealed his story.

He had always been a rather solitary man, who lived alone and had few close friends and no close family members in the city. In his late thirties he met a woman, fell in love, and married. He described his wife as a lovely and gracious woman, also from Europe, a devoted homemaker who had agreed to his request that they have no children so that she might attend only to him.

Shortly after his retirement, 6 years prior to his coming to seek help, on their first visit to Europe, WW was confronted by his wife's deficits in memory and orientation. Years of many consultations with several physicians followed. Mrs. WW's Alzheimer's disease (diagnosed with full general medical and neurological workups) progressed steadily. She gradually became no longer able to recognize her husband and to need total care. She had been in several good nursing homes during the previous 3 years. Most but not all of the family's financial assets and savings had been spent on her care.

WW was devoted to his wife's condition and care. He spent every day with her in the nursing home, feeding her each meal himself and bringing frequent gifts to the staff members, especially nurses, certain they would not care for his wife unless "bribed" in this way.

He was chronically bitterly enraged at all medical and social service workers for their inadequacies in the face of his wife's illness. He would not acknowledge his anger, but expressed it so clearly through his demeaning, sarcastic yet superficially ingratiating behavior that many people responded poorly to him. He often felt lonely and discouraged, feelings that were minimally relieved by rare social visits with the few relatives he and his wife had.

As a precipitant to this visit, WW had received a distressing phone call regarding his application for Medicaid for his wife. He was asked detailed questions about his remaining finances, and it became clear that Medicaid would be denied. Following the call, he had the sudden onset of visual problems (blurry vision, dizziness, "spots") and came to the emergency room several days later where his ophthalmologic exam was normal. A review of his hospital chart revealed a history of several years of clinic and emergency room visits for various physical complaints (e.g., hearing or visual complaint, chest or gastrointestinal pain, flat feet) with little organic etiology found. His frequent visits and occasional tearful behavior would elicit social service referrals, but WW would refuse outright or just not follow up with appointments or groups. On questioning, he admitted to belonging to the largest support group for spouses of Alzheimer patients, but commented, "I'll only go when they get a cure."

Remaining aspects of the mental status exam showed normal speech with no psychomotor retardation or agitation and no prominent vegetative signs. His affect was full-range but mildly suspicious and easily angered. He denied suicidal or homicidal ideation or intent, excusing his earlier statements as jokes and something he would never be able to do. He had no gross thought disorder, but did exhibit paranoid trends in his thinking, e.g., comparing the emergency room to being "in prison." Cognitive functioning was excellent.

After opening up to tell his story, WW again became angry and devaluing and refused any further help or discussion. We empathized with the difficulties of his situation, spoke to him about the risk of depression, and, given that he refused all other recommendations, invited him to return to the psychiatric emergency room to speak with staff there at any time.

Discussion

This case demonstrates the difficulties in forming a therapeutic alliance with a family member who cannot see himself as a designated patient and who rejects the very support and assistance he needs (and perhaps asks for with his somatic complaints, "joking" remarks, and troubling behavior). In WW, we see a familiar constellation of problems in spouses of AD patients: anger, isolation, the interplay of stress and underlying character traits and disorders, and the financial strain of chronic illness. WW's unwillingness to accept therapy illustrates the challenge of how to help those who are at the same time in need, at risk, and reluctant.

CASE EXAMPLE 9

Key Clinical Issues

Alzheimer's disease with delusions
Problem behaviors in AD
AD with compounding physical illness
AD patient with mentally ill spouse
Hospitalization for the AD patient
AD patients and disposition problems

The Case

A frantic phone call to a psychiatrist by the daughter of an elderly couple, Mr. and Mrs. DG, resulted in the daughter being seen that afternoon. During the interview, the daughter clearly defined the problem. Her mother, 72 years old, a chronic schizophrenic, had been maintained at home by her father for the past 20 years. Her father, now 80 years old, had been gradually deteriorating physically and mentally during the past five years.

However, within the past year the mother had been complaining to her married, pregnant daughter that her father had been molesting her sexually and exposing himself in the neighborhood. The daughter's immediate reaction was "Well, mother is delusional and hallucinating again." However, when these complaints persisted, the daughter asked some of the neighbors if there was any truth to the accusations, and to her surprise some of them were affirmed. She then began to visit her parents on a daily basis and noted that her father was talking to himself, very forgetful, very suspicious of her and the neighbors, and at times misidentified her. On one occasion she walked into her parents' home and saw her naked father literally chasing her mother around the rooms.

It was at that point she made the decision to do something and asked for the consultation. When she was told that it sounded as if her father had to be hospitalized, she immediately responded, "It will kill my mother." Yet she acknowledged that an appropriate support system was not available and that she herself, 7 months pregnant with a 2-year-old child at home, could not continue at the present pace. She agreed to have her father hospitalized.

At the hospital he was noted to have uncontrolled diabetes mellitus as part of his clinical problems. During the initial stages of the hospitalization, he was observed on a number of different occasions to expose himself to female patients, while expressing paranoid ideas in a hostile, suspicious manner. When the diabetes was controlled, he was started on small doses of an antipsychotic. His suspiciousness subsided, as well as his belligerence and sexual indiscretions. A comprehensive examination led to a diagnosis, in addition to the diabetes, of Alzheimer's disease. At this point the mother was hospitalized on the same unit because of increasing agitation, insomnia, delusions, and hallucinations. When she saw her husband, her delusions about her husband being murdered subsided. However, she subsequently needed regulation of her antipsychotic medications. By this time both she and her husband were discharged as a couple to a nearby long-term care facility.

Discussion

Because Alzheimer's disease is mostly a disorder of later life, it can be compounded by physical illness, which is more likely in the elderly. When treated successfully for the physical illness, the symptoms which can be attributed to AD may subside. This represents yet another source of excess disability in these patients.

The concept of the "second patient" in Alzheimer's disease is also addressed here. While there is growing attention to the risk of a caregiver developing a reactive depression when confronted with the burdens of care, less focus has been placed on the added complexity of the primary caregiver already having a serious illness.

CASE EXAMPLE 10

Key Clinical Issues

The clinical phenomenon of pseudodementia, with attention to diagnosis and differential diagnosis.

The First Meeting

RF was a 78-year-old man, a retired physician who lived with his wife in a fashionable residential area. The patient had recently been hospitalized at a VA hospital for treatment of multiple medical problems and evaluation of apparent dementia. Nursing home placement was planned, but the patient was transferred to the geropsychiatry inpatient service for evaluation of worsening depression.

RF was accompanied by his wife to the ward. The history was obtained from them conjointly. When he first came on the ward, the patient sat stooped in his wheelchair. He spoke very slowly in muted tones. He declined to answer most questions, frequently saying, "I can't remember," or, "I don't care about that," in response. After much coaxing, he stated that he started losing his health and his mind 9 years earlier, and that his poor health had caused him to retire. The patient reported having had a pacemaker implanted at that time because of severe arrhythmias. Nonetheless, he had continued his practice until he began having much more difficulty with his memory, aggravated further by greatly diminished energy. He stated that he was told that all of these symptoms resulted from his heart disease. His wife interrupted, saying that his heart disease was actually well controlled and it was unclear why he had retired. RF became angry at this point. He raised the tone of his voice and said, "You are always pushing me to do more; you never let me rest even though I am sick. You think you know better? Fine, you tell the doctor!" His wife then proceeded with the history, her statements punctuated by her husband's muttering, "Oh, she's crazy," or "What does she want from me?"

She stated that her husband was "always overreacting to his illness" and had never adjusted to having heart disease. She felt that he had "given up" by retiring, and that although he had started to experience memory problems, they were not severe. Still, he did get some enjoyment in his retirement from reading books, keeping up with his journals, and traveling with her. Approximately 2 years after his retirment, RF was diagnosed as having hypothyroidism for which he was started on levothyroxine. He monitored the dose himself, refusing to see a physician. One year later, he developed mild parkinsonism for which he was treated with carbidopa-levodopa by a neurologist. Throughout the first 8 years of his retirement, RF developed gradually worsening congestive heart failure for which he was treated with various diuretics, digoxin, and most recently propranolol.

RF's wife stated that he "always had problems" accepting these illnesses and commented that he would soon "rot away." At the same time, she allowed that he had done fairly well until a year ago, when she noted him becoming increasingly depressed and withdrawn. He had considerably less interest in going out and just wanted to watch television.

Approximately 5 months before admission, RF was involved in an automobile accident in which his car was severely damaged by an uninsured motorist from whom he could collect no compensation.

Although the patient suffered no bodily harm, his wife reported that his mood and cognition deteriorated markedly at that time. He constantly complained of being weak and fatigued and completely stopped reading his journals. She said he appeared quite confused and disoriented at times. RF complained of increasing dizziness and slowly "seemed to lose the ability to walk." He slept more than usual, napping frequently during the day, but his weight and appetite remained unchanged.

RF was admitted to a community medical hospital because of his problems functioning at home. He had an extensive medical and neurologic workup which revealed a new finding of hypercalcemia. A parathyroid adenoma was diagnosed, but this condition was not judged severe enough to treat. The parkinsonism medication was discontinued because of possible contribution to his declining mental status. Throughout the hospitalization, RF was found to be poorly oriented to place and time with poor short- and long-term memory. He was noted to be moderately depressed, but his physicians concluded that this was probably a reaction to his declining mental status.

RF did not improve during this hospitalization. He was hospitalized on several additional occasions for numerous somatic complaints for which no treatment was given. During the last hospitalization, he was given a diagnosis of "organic mental depression," and his wife was told that nothing more could be done for him. She was informed that if his condition continued to deteriorate, he might have to be placed in a nursing home. When his deterioration continued, she had him admitted to the VA because she felt he was "no longer welcome at the other hospital."

The family history revealed that the patient and his wife had been married for 53 years. They had two children who were both in their 30s. Their son lived in town, but the parents were not in close contact with either child. The social history revealed that the patient and his wife had never spent very much time together until his retirement. She had raised their children and taken care of the house. RF had started his practice in a small town in the Midwest where he had been successful and highly regarded. He had always been involved in his practice. They subsequently moved to the West Coast where RF became Chief of Medicine at a large hospital, remaining in that position for the next 25 years until his retirement. They had some difficulties in their relationship around the time of his retirement, but after 2 years were getting along well. She had maintained her interests, activities, and friends outside of the house, whereas he led a more solitary life.

The two of them were not well prepared financially for retirement. RF's position was prestigious and they were financially comfortable while he worked, but his pension was small and they had not saved much. They had had to reduce their standard of living noticeably after he retired. The loss of their car in the accident had placed an additional financial burden on them.

The mental status exam revealed RF to be apathetic and withdrawn. He knew that he was in a hospital, but did not know the date or why he was there. His speech was slowed, he made little eye contact, and he had significant psychomotor retardation. His mood was depressed and his affect was flattened. His attention and concentration were impaired as assessed by his limited digit span and ability to perform serial subtraction. With considerable urging and encouragement, however, his calculations and abstract reasoning were good. Although he spoke slowly and used few words, his vocabulary was good. He refused testing of his visuospatial skills.

The physical examination revealed RF to be wasted and moderately dehydrated. He had moderately severe symptoms of Parkinson's disease with marked stiffness and bradykinesia. There were no signs of congestive heart failure, and the rest of the physical exam was normal.

Approach to Diagnosis

The patient presented a complicated picture with apparent cognitive losses and multiple medical problems, being treated with medications, as well as signs of depression. The patient's pattern of cognitive loss was not characteristic of a dementing process, however. Many of his apparent deficits were secondary to poor motivation or inattentiveness. Furthermore, his deficits were spotty and some spheres of function, such as language, seemed relatively intact. Therefore, despite the magnitude of the patient's disability, the primary disease process was unlikely to be dementia.

The patient appeared to have significant signs and symptoms of depression. The patient certainly had multiple stressors and life changes, as well as physical illnesses, that could contribute to depression. In addition, the patient was taking medications that could precipitate or exacerbate depression, and the patient's Parkinson's disease could make him appear more depressed than he really was.

Given the mood, affect, neurovegetative signs, and cognitive impairment, a major depressive episode was the most likely diagnosis in this case.

Treatment

Starting antidepressant medication was considered. Given the number of medical problems in his case, however, it was decided first to evaluate and treat these disorders. Furthermore, given the number of stressors that the patient had suffered, as well as his history of not coping well with physical illness, supportive psychotherapy seemed indicated.

The patient was started back on his parkinsonism medication, and the dosage was gradually increased. Within a few days of hospitalization and this medication change, RF was brighter and more active. His psychomotor retardation lessened and his concentration improved. His mood was persistently depressed, however, and he began to cry more easily.

The patient's propranolol was stopped because of a possible contribution to his depression and was replaced with a diuretic. At this point, the patient's thyroid function test results were reported revealing low T_3 and T_4 and slightly elevated TSH. Levothyroxine dosages were therefore gradually increased. The patient's serum calcium was slightly elevated, but this was not judged to be significant enough to treat.

Clinical Course

Over the first week of hospitalization, RF's mood and affect gradually improved. He remained aloof from most of the staff and patients and seemed disdainful of his psychiatrist. As his cognitive status improved, he began to question his psychiatrist incessantly about the treatment and, in the view of the therapist, seemed determined to prove that he was not doing a good job.

RF began to express his feelings of anger more directly in therapy. He was confronted with his behavior toward his physician and the ward staff and was able to recognize his actions as manifestations of his anger. RF began to express some feelings of bitterness and then of sadness regarding his retirement 9 years earlier. He revealed that he had felt "pushed out" by the younger physicians, with whom he had felt he could not compete, especially due to his failing memory. His therapist, who was a resident, observed that RF probably felt anger at him because he was much younger and just starting his career. The patient responded positively to this observation, and subsequently was less angry and more open with his therapist.

The therapy then focused more on the stresses that the patient had suffered in the year immediately prior to the hospitalization, particularly his automobile accident. RF at first denied that this event had any significance to him beyond having caused him anger and inconvenience. As the topic was explored, however, RF was able to express the tremendous feelings of helplessness with which his accident had left him. The accident seemed to highlight for him the loss of control that he felt about his life, and that he was ruled by circumstances beyond his control. The patient had strong associations to the feelings that he had felt when he learned of each of his illnesses, over which he also felt powerless.

RF improved throughout a 4-week hospitalization to the extent that he was able to perform his own activities of daily living. His mood and affect were much improved; his wife remarked, "He hasn't looked this good in three years." During the last week of hospitalization, two conjoint meetings were held. The patient had feared these meetings and regressed somewhat as his wife began to express anger at his behavior over the last year. But by the end of the second meeting, the wife made clear her happiness at RF's improvement and that she wanted him to come home.

The patient was discharged from the hospital, but continued for 3 months in weekly psychotherapy with another psychiatrist. The therapy was reported to focus on helping the patient to learn to live within the limits imposed by his circumstances. His sense of control over his life was enhanced by identifying those interests of his that he could pursue. Psychological testing was obtained, which demonstrated that the patient was largely cognitively intact with only mild memory loss. This report was shared with the patient, and it seemed to encourage him considerably.

Discussion

While pseudodementia has been more classically seen as depression masquerading as dementia, other factors such as drug toxicity and physical illness may contribute to its manifestation.

This case illustrates the importance of distinguishing pseudodementia from Alzheimer's disease. While there can be confusing surface similarities, pseudodementia can be cleared up and the patient's overall level of functioning significantly improved and stabilized.

REFERENCE

American Psychiatric Association (1987). *Diagnostic and statistical manual of mental disorders* (3rd ed. rev.). Washington, DC: APA.

6
CONCLUSION

Eighty years after Alzheimer's classic case was published in 1907, a National Institutes of Health Consensus Development Statement (1987), *Differential Diagnosis of Dementing Disorders,* emphasized that "dementia is primarily a behavioral diagnosis." For most of those 8 decades the interest in Alzheimer's disease had come mostly from the research sector, with the predominant attention focused on the intriguing neuropathology of the disorder— particularly the plaques and tangles that were described in the original paper. But the original paper also described a clinical picture that pointed the direction toward clinical intervention and the role of service providers, namely, the opportunity to treat excess disability caused by behavioral symptomatology and family stress. An understanding of the behavioral dysfunction and psychosocial complications that accompany this brain disorder and an awareness of how to treat the excess disability aspects of these problems are among the major contributions of psychiatric skill in the overall approach to Alzheimer's disease.

REFERENCE

National Institutes of Health Consensus Development Statement. (1987, July 6–8). *Differential diagnosis of dementing diseases, 6*(11).

BIBLIOGRAPHY

BRIEF OVERVIEWS

Cohen, G.D. (1987). Alzheimer's disease. In G. L. Maddox (Ed.), *Encyclopedia of Aging* (pp. 27–30). New York: Springer.

Katzman, R. (1986). Alzheimer's disease. *New England Journal of Medicine, 31*(13), 964–973.

Wurtman, R.J. (1985). Alzheimer's disease. *Scientific American, 252*(1), 62–74.

IN-DEPTH REVIEWS

Strong on Both Basic Science and Clinical Issues

Reisberg, B. (Ed.). (1983). *Alzheimer's disease.* New York: Free Press.

Strong on Clinical and Policy Issues

Gilhooly, L.M., Zarit, S.H., & Birren, J.E. (Eds.). (1986). *The dementias: Policy and management.* Englewood Cliffs, NJ: Prentice-Hall.

Miller, N.E., & Cohen, G.D. (Eds.). (1981). *Clinical aspects of Alzheimer's disease and senile dementia.* New York: Raven Press.

Strong on Basic Science

Katzman, R., Terry, R.D., & Bick, K.L. (Eds.). (1978). *Alzheimer's disease: senile dementia and related disorders.* New York: Raven Press.

Katzman, R. (Ed.). (1983). *Biological aspects of Alzheimer's disease.* Cold Spring Harbor Laboratory, NY: Banbury Reports.

Broad Overview (Epidemiology, Research, Services, Financing, Policy)

US Congress, Office of Technology Assessment. (1987). *Losing a million minds. Confronting the tragedy of Alzheimer's disease and other dementias.* Washington, DC: US Government Printing Office (OTA-BA-323).

Family References

Cohen, D., & Eisdorfer, C. (1986). *The loss of self.* New York: Norton.
Mace, N.L., & Rabins, P.V. (1981). *The 36-hour day.* Baltimore: Johns Hopkins University Press.

JOURNAL

Alzheimer's Disease and Associated Disorders, S.S. Matsuyama & L.F. Jarvik (Eds.). Lawrence, KS: Western Geriatric Research Institute. The Journal contains regular articles plus abstracts of articles on Alzheimer's disease from other journals and books.

APPENDIX: RATING SCALES

NOTE: Administration of these tests may be technically difficult under certain circumstances; accordingly, we recommend reviewing the specific guidelines given for them in the references cited.

INTRODUCTION

A variety of rating scales are available for assessing different parameters, including cognition, affect, behavior, etc. These are frequently utilized in research studies but have not been incorporated as readily into the daily routine clinical evaluation of patients. This is unfortunate since these scales objectify findings and many of them may be used to follow the course of a patient longitudinally. The scales referred to here are not the only acceptable ones available, but are the ones frequently utilized by researchers and clinicians, or have been validated for the specific patient population. For example, although the Hamilton Depression Scale has been used frequently in geriatric depression studies, it has not been incorporated here since it is not specific to this age population. On the other hand, the Yesavage Depression Rating Scale has been validated in this age group.

Other scales such as the Mini Mental State Exam are used frequently. Frequent use, however, does not necessarily imply that they are free of problems. For example, the Mini Mental State Exam cannot be used with any degree of validity with individuals uneducated or alien to this country when questions are specifically geared to political events or situations of this country. Furthermore, it is not sensitive enough to identify patients accurately in the very early stages of dementia. Although these scales are not ideal or necessarily diagnostic, they nonetheless add another dimension to the clinical diagnosis and monitoring of the progression of the illness.

MINI MENTAL STATE EXAM

Score   Orientation

( )   What is the (year) (season) (month) (date) (day)? (5 points)
( )   Where are we? (state) (county) (town) (hospital) (floor) (5 points)

Registration

( )   Name 3 objects: 1 second to say each. Then ask the patient to repeat all three after you have said them. 1 point for each correct. Then repeat them until he learns them. Record, too, the number of repetitions you provide. (3 points)

Attention and Calculation

( )   Serial 7s. (subtract 7 from 100, then 7 from that answer, etc.) 1 point for each correct. Stop at 5 answers. Or spell "world" backwards. (Number correct = letters before mistake, i.e., d l o r w = 2 correct). (5 points)

Recall

( )   Ask for the objects above. 1 point for each correct. (3 points)

Language Tests

( )   Identify by name: pencil, watch (2 points)
( )   Repeat: "No ifs, ands or buts" (1 point)
( )   Follow a 3-stage command: "Take the paper in your right hand, fold it in half, and put it on the floor." (3 points)

Read and obey the following

( )   Close your eyes. (1 point)
( )   Write a sentence spontaneously below. (1 point)

( )   Copy design below. (1 point)

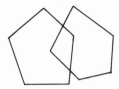

( )   Total 30 points

Scoring

Score of 25 or greater—considered normal.
Score of 20 or less—suggests the presence of dementia.

See Folstein, Folstein & McHugh, 1975

BLESSED DEMENTIA SCALE

Changes in Performance of Everyday Activities

1. Inability to perform household tasks   1 ½ 0
2. Inability to cope with small sums of money   1 ½ 0
3. Inability to remember short list of items, e.g., in
   shopping   1 ½ 0
4. Inability to find way about indoors   1 ½ 0
5. Inability to find way about familiar streets   1 ½ 0
6. Inability to interpret surroundings (e.g., to recognize
   whether in hospital, or at home, to discriminate
   between patients, doctors and nurses, relatives and
   hosptial staff, etc.)   1 ½ 0
7. Inability to recall recent events (e.g., recent outings,
   visits of relatives or friends to hospital, etc.)   1 ½ 0
8. Tendency to dwell in the past   1 ½ 0

Changes in Habits

9. Eating:
   Cleanly with proper utensils   0
   Messily with spoon only   2
   Simple solids, e.g., biscuits   2
   Has to be fed   3
10. Dressing:
    Unaided   0
    Occasionally misplaced buttons, etc.   1
    Wrong sequence, commonly forgetting items   2
    Unable to dress   3
11. Complete sphincter control   0
    Occasional wet beds   1
    Frequent wet beds   2
    Double incontinent   3

Changes in Personality, Interests, Drive

	No change	0
12.	Increased rigidity	1
13.	Increased egocentricity	1
14.	Impairment of regard for feelings of others	1
15.	Coarsening of affect	1
16.	Impairment of emotional control, e.g., increased petulance and irritability	1
17.	Hilarity in inappropriate situations	1
18.	Diminished emotional responsiveness	1
19.	Sexual misdemeanor (appearing *de novo* in old age)	1
	Interests retained	0
20.	Hobbies relinquished	1
21.	Diminished initiative or growing apathy	1
22.	Purposeless hyperactivity	1

Total _____

Scoring

Score of 4 or less—little or no deterioration of cognitive function
Score of 5 or greater—consistent with definite and marked cognitive deficts

See Blessed, Tomlinson & Roth, 1968

HACHINSKI ISCHEMIC SCALE

---

1. Onset of symptoms was abrupt   (2)_____
2. Stepwise deterioration   (1)_____
3. Fluctuating course (returns to near normal func-   (2)_____
   tion for a day or more at a time
4. Nocturnal confusion (score only if symptoms are   (1)_____
   essentially confined to the night hours)
5. Relative preservation of personality   (1)_____
6. Depression   (1)_____
7. Somatic complaints   (1)_____
8. Emotional incontinence   (1)_____
9. History of hypertension   (1)_____
10. History of strokes (family was told by a physician   (2)_____
    that the patient had had a stroke)
11. Evidence of associated atherosclerosis (EKG, chest   (1)_____
    x-ray, pulse deficits, etc.)
12. Focal neurological symptoms   (2)_____
13. Focal neurological signs   (2)_____

Total: (0–18)_____

Scoring

Total score of 7 and above—consistent with a diagnosis of multi-
infarct dementia

Score of 4 or less—suggestive of primary degenerative dementia

---

See Hachinski, Lassen & Marshall, 1974

GERIATRIC DEPRESSION SCALE

Choose the best answer for how you felt over the past week

1. Are you basically satisfied with your life?   yes/no
2. Have you dropped many of your activities and interests?   yes/no
3. Do you feel that your life is empty?   yes/no
4. Do you often get bored?   yes/no
5. Are you hopeful about the future?   yes/no
6. Are you bothered by thoughts you can't get out of your head?   yes/no
7. Are you in good spirits most of the time?   yes/no
8. Are you afraid that something is going to happen to you?   yes/no
9. Do you feel happy most of the time?   yes/no
10. Do you often feel helpless?   yes/no
11. Do you often get restless and fidgety?   yes/no
12. Do you prefer to stay home, rather than going out and doing new things?   yes/no
13. Do you frequently worry about the future?   yes/no
14. Do you feel you have more problems with memory than most?   yes/no
15. Do you think it is wonderful to be alive now?   yes/no
16. Do you often feel downhearted and blue?   yes/no
17. Do you feel pretty worthless the way you are now?   yes/no
18. Do you worry a lot about the past?   yes/no
19. Do you find life very exciting?   yes/no
20. Is it hard for you to get started on new projects?   yes/no
21. Do you feel full of energy?   yes/no
22. Do you feel that your situation is hopeless?   yes/no
23. Do you think that most people are better off than you are?   yes/no
24. Do you frequently get upset over little things?   yes/no
25. Do you frequently feel like crying?   yes/no
26. Do you have trouble concentrating?   yes/no
27. Do you enjoy getting up in the mornings?   yes/no
28. Do you prefer to avoid social gatherings?   yes/no
29. Is it easy for you to make decisions?   yes/no
30. Is your mind as clear as it used to be?   yes/no

Scoring

Of the 30 questions, 20 indicate the presence of depression when answered positively, with each positive response receiving one point. The other 10 questions, (1, 5, 7, 9, 15, 19, 21, 27, 29, 30) indicate depression when answered negatively, each negative response receiving one point.

Total score of 5 or less—considered normal
Score of 15 to 21—signifies mild depression
Score of 22 or higher—consistent with severe depression

See Yesavage et al., 1983

DEMENTIA BEHAVIOR SCALE

Name: _____ Date: _____

Total: _____ Rater's Initials: _____

Language/Conversation

0 Conversational
1 Repeats self, searches for synonyms, reticent conversation
2 Circumlocution, white lies, mild vocabulary limitation, easily led in conversation, automatisms
3 Loses thread of thought, noticeable vocabulary loss
4 Less aware of mistakes, poor syntax and sequence, perseveration, neologisms
5 Parrots words, incoherent, uncomprehending, severe vocabulary limitation
6 Mute, unresponsive

Social Interaction

0 Assists, takes initiative
1 Active participant, follower
2 Bland participant, no longer empathic, loss of tact, withdrawn, clinging
3 Observer only, misidentifies close relatives, at times belligerent/ defensive/suspicious
4 Out of step, poor recognition of persons, mistakes own reflection, at times menacing
5 Wanders, frequent catastrophic reaction (defiant, suspicious, combative)
6 Blank

Attention/Awareness

0 Bright, responsive
1 Requires guidance, can't recall date
2 Shortened attention, can't recall day, easily distracted
3 Wandering attention, easily tires, very few pleasures
4 Distracted by illusions, picks at imaginary lint, misidentifies objects
5 Can be engaged sporadically and briefly
6 Oblivious

Spatial Orientation

0 Oriented
1 Oriented to immediate locus only (can't get home)
2 Hesitant, loses things
3 Disoriented to place, hides things, pack rat
4 Body disorientations, can't seat self on chair, bodily illusions, oblivious to posture
5 Hallucinating
6 Totally lost

Motor Coordination

0 Fully coordinated
1 Underactive, responsive to commands
2 Poorly coordinated, slowly moving, stumbling
3 Occasionally requires manipulation, occasionally requires assistance
4 Involuntary movements interfere, immobile, neglect of one side, requires manipulation and assistance
5 Spastic, chin on chest, wheelchair for safety, maximum physical assistance
6 Unable to ambulate, limbs contracted

Bowel and Bladder

0   Self-care
1   Asks to go, needs clues to locate toilet
2   Remindable, poor hygiene occasionally, forgets to flush
3   Regular supervision, requires assistance, occasionally wet
4   Occasional fecal incontinence
5   Unpredictable, control by enema, occasional diapers
6   Fully incontinent, full-time diapers, full-time catheter

Eating and Nutrition

0   Self-care, weight steady, can cook
1   Needs prompting to eat, history of weight loss, burns pots
2   Needs food cut up, wanders from table, can't cook at all
3   Improper use of utensils, uses fingers, slight weight gain
4   Voraciously interested in sweets, steals food, marked weight gain, marked weight loss
5   Must be fed, eats nonfood
6   Tube fed, dysphagic

Dress and Grooming

0   Appropriate self-care, well groomed
1   Won't change, poorly groomed
2   Dirty, ill-kempt, inappropriate dress, food on face
3   Misuse of clothing, misidentification of clothes, wears other's clothes, needs clothes set out
4   Dresses with instructions and help, oblivious to grooming
5   Requires full assistance
6   Must be dressed, hospital gown

Scoring

Score of 9 or less—normal
Score of 10 or more—consistent with a dementia

From Haycox (1984). Reprinted by permission from *The Journal of Clinical Psychiatry*.

REFERENCES

Blessed, G., Tomlinson, B.E., & Roth, M. (1968). The association between quantitative mesures of dementia and of senile change in the cerebral grey matter of elderly subjects. *British Journal of Psychiatry, 114,* 797–811.

Folstein, M., Folstein, S., & McHugh, P.R. (1975). Mini-mental state: A practical method of grading the cognitive state of patients for the clinician. *Journal of Psychiatric Research, 12,* 189–198.

Hachinski, V.C., Lassen, N.A., & Marshall, J. (1974). Multi-infarct dementia: A cause of mental deterioration in the elderly. *Lancet, 2,* 207–209.

Haycox, J.A. (1984). The Dementia Behavior Scale. *Journal of Clinical Psychiatry, 45,* 23–24.

Yesavage, J.A., Brink, T.L., Rose, T.J., et al. (1983). Development and validation of a geriatric depression screening scale: A preliminary report. *Journal of Psychiatric Research, 17,* 37–49.

INDEX

GAP COMMITTEES AND MEMBERSHIP

COMMITTEE ON ADOLESCENCE
Clarice J. Kestenbaum, New York, NY,
  Chairperson
Hector R. Bird, New York, NY
Ian A. Canino, New York, NY
Warren J. Gadpaille, Denver, CO
Michael G. Kalogerakis, New York, NY
Silvio J. Onesti, Jr., Belmont, MA

COMMITTEE ON ALCOHOLISM AND THE
  ADDICTIONS
Edward J. Khantzian, Haverhill, MA,
  Chairperson
Margaret H. Bean-Bayog, Lexington,
  MA
Richard J. Frances, Newark, NJ
Sheldon I. Miller, Newark, NJ
Robert B. Millman, New York, NY
Steven M. Mirin, Westwood, MA
Edgar P. Nace, Dallas, TX
Norman L. Paul, Lexington, MA
Peter Steinglass, Washington, DC
John S. Tamerin, Greenwich, CT

COMMITTEE ON CHILD PSYCHIATRY
Theodore Shapiro, New York, NY,
  Chairperson
James M. Bell, Canaan, NY
Harlow Donald Dunton, New York, NY
Joseph Fischhoff, Detroit, MI
Joseph M. Green, Madison, WI
John F. McDermott, Jr., Honolulu, HI
John Schowalter, New Haven, CT
Peter E. Tanguay, Los Angeles, CA
Lenore Terr, San Francisco, CA

COMMITTEE ON COLLEGE STUDENTS
Myron B. Liptzin, Chapel Hill, NC,
  Chairperson
Robert L. Arnstein, Hamden, CT
Varda Backus, La Jolla, CA
Harrison P. Eddy, New York, NY
Malkah Tolpin Notman, Brookline,
  MA
Gloria C. Onque, Pittsburgh, PA
Elizabeth Aub Reid, Cambridge, MA
Earle Silber, Chevy Chase, MD
Tom G. Stauffer, White Plains, NY

COMMITTEE ON CULTURAL PSYCHIATRY
Ezra E.H. Griffith, New Haven, CT,
  Chairperson
Edward F. Foulks, New Orleans, LA
Pedro Ruiz, Houston, TX
John P. Spiegel, Waltham, MA
Ronald M. Wintrob, Providence, RI
Joe Yamamoto, Los Angeles, CA

COMMITTEE ON THE FAMILY
Herta A. Guttman, Montreal, Quebec,
  Chairperson
W. Robert Beavers, Dallas, TX
Ellen M. Berman, Merrion, PA
Lee Combrinck-Graham, Evanston, IL
Ira D. Glick, New York, NY
Frederick Gottlieb, Los Angeles, CA
Henry U. Grunebaum, Cambridge,
  MA
Judith Landau-Stanton, Rochester, NY
Ann L. Price, Hartford, CT
Lyman C. Wynne, Rochester, NY

155

Stanley I. Greenspan, Bethesda, MD
Harris B. Peck, New Rochelle, NY
Naomi Rae-Grant, Hamilton, Ontario
Morton M. Silverman, Bethesda, MD
Anne Marie Wolf-Schatz,
  Conshohocken, PA

COMMITTEE ON PUBLIC EDUCATION
Keith H. Johansen, Dallas, TX,
  Chairperson
Susan J. Blumenthal, Washington, DC
Jack W. Bonner, III, Asheville, NY
Steven E. Katz, New York, NY
Boris G. Rifkin, Branford, CT
Robert A. Solow, Los Angeles, CA
Calvin R. Sumner, Buckhannon, WV
Kenneth N. Vogtsberger, San Antonio,
  TX

COMMITTEE ON PSYCHIATRY AND THE
  COMMUNITY
Kenneth Minkoff, Woburn, MA,
  Chairperson
C. Knight Aldrich, Charlottesville, VA
David G. Greenfield, Guilford, CT
H. Richard Lamb, Los Angeles, CA
John C. Nemiah, Hanover, NH
Rebecca L. Potter, Tucson, AZ
Alexander S. Rogawski, Los Angeles,
  CA
John J. Schwab, Louisville, KY
John A. Talbott, Baltimore, MD
Charles B. Wilkinson, Kansas City, MO

COMMITTEE ON PSYCHIATRY AND LAW
Jonas R. Rappeport, Baltimore, MD,
  Chairperson
Park E. Dietz, Charlottesville, VA
John Donnelly, Hartford, CT
Carl P. Malmquist, Minneapolis, MN
Herbert C. Modlin, Topeka, KS
Phillip J. Resnick, Cleveland, OH
Loren H. Roth, Pittsburgh, PA

Joseph Satten, San Francisco, CA
William D. Weitzel, Lexington, KY
Howard V. Zonana, New Haven, CT

COMMITTEE ON PSYCHIATRY AND
  RELIGION
Albert J. Lubin, Woodside, CA,
  Chairperson
Sidney Furst, Bronx, NY
Richard C. Lewis, New Haven, CT
Earl A. Loomis, Jr., Augusta, GA
Abigail R. Ostow, Belmont, MA
Mortimer Ostow, Bronx, NY
Sally K. Severino, White Plains, NY
Clyde R. Snyder, Fayetteville, NC

COMMITTEE ON PSYCHIATRY IN INDUSTRY
Barrie S. Greiff, Cambridge, MA,
  Chairperson
Peter L. Brill, Radnor, PA
Duane Q. Hagen, St. Louis, MO
R. Edward Huffman, Asheville, NC
David E. Morrison, Palatine, IL
David B. Robbins, Chappaqua, NY
Jay B. Rohrlich, New York, NY
Clarence J. Rowe, St. Paul, MN
Jeffrey L. Speller, Alexandria, VA

COMMITTEE ON PSYCHOPATHOLOGY
David A. Adler, Boston, MA,
  Chairperson
Jeffrey Berlant, Summit, NJ
Robert E. Drake, Hanover, NH
James M. Ellison, Watertown, MA
Howard H. Goldman, Rockville, MD
Richard E. Renneker, Los Angeles, CA

COMMITTEE ON RESEARCH
Robert Cancro, New York, NY,
  Chairperson
Kenneth Z. Altshuler, Dallas, TX
Jack A. Grebb, New York, NY

John H. Greist, Madison, WI
Jerry M. Lewis, Dallas, TX
Morris A. Lipton, Chapel Hill, NC
John G. Looney, Durham, NC
Sidney Malitz, New York, NY
Zebulon Taintor, Orangeburg, NY

COMMITTEE ON SOCIAL ISSUES
Ian E. Alger, New York, NY, Chairperson
William R. Beardslee, Boston, MA
Judith H. Gold, Halifax, Nova Scotia
Roderic Gorney, Los Angeles, CA
Martha J. Kirkpatrick, Los Angeles, CA
Perry Ottenberg, Philadelphia, PA
Kendon W. Smith, Piermont, NY

COMMITTEE ON THERAPEUTIC CARE
Donald W. Hammersley, Bethesda, MD, Chairperson
Bernard Bandler, Cambridge, MA
Thomas E. Curtis, Chapel Hill, NC
William B. Hunter, III, Albuquerque, NM
Roberto L. Jimenez, San Antonio, TX
Milton Kramer, Cincinnati, OH
Theodore Nadelson, Jamaica Plain, MA
William W. Richards, Anchorage, AK

COMMITTEE ON THERAPY
Allen D. Rosenblatt, La Jolla, CA, Chairperson
Jules R. Bemporad, Boston, MA
Henry W. Brosin, Tucson, AZ
Eugene B. Feigelson, Brooklyn, NY
Robert Michels, New York, NY
Andrew P. Morrison, Cambridge, MA
William C. Offenkrantz, Carefree, AZ

CONTRIBUTING MEMBERS
John E. Adams, Gainesville, FL
Carlos C. Alden, Jr., Buffalo, NY
Spencer Bayles, Houston, TX
C. Christian Beels, New York, NY
Elissa P. Benedek, Ann Arbor, MI
Sidney Berman, Washington, DC
H. Keith H. Brodie, Durham, NC
Charles M. Bryant, San Francisco, CA
Ewald W. Busse, Durham, NC
Robert N. Butler, New York, NY
Eugene M. Caffey, Jr., Bowie, MD
Ian L.W. Clancey, Maitland, Ontario
Sanford I. Cohen, Boston, MA
James S. Eaton, Jr., Washington, DC
Lloyd C. Elam, Nashville, TN
Stanley H. Eldred, Belmont, MA
Joseph T. English, New York, NY
Louis C. English, Pomona, NY
Sherman C. Feinstein, Highland Park, IL
Archie R. Foley, New York, NY
Henry J. Gault, Highland Park, IL
Alexander Gralnick, Port Chester, NY
Milton Greenblatt, Sylmar, CA
Lawrence F. Greenleigh, Los Angeles, CA
Jon E. Gudeman, Milwaukee, WI
Stanley Hammons, Lexington, KY
William Hetznecker, Merion Station, PA
J. Cotter Hirschberg, Topeka, KS
Jay Katz, New Haven, CT
James A. Knight, New Orleans, LA
Othilda M. Krug, Cincinnati, OH
Alan I. Levenson, Tucson, AZ
Ruth W. Lidz, Woodbridge, CT
Orlando B. Lightfoot, Boston, MA
Reginald S. Lourie, Chevy Chase, MD
Norman L. Loux, Sellersville, PA
John A. MacLeod, Cincinnati, OH
Leo Madow, Philadelphia, PA
Charles A. Malone, Barrington, RI
Peter A. Martin, Lake Orion, MI
Ake Mattsson, Danderyd, Sweden
Alan A. McLean, Westport, CT
David Mendell, Houston, TX

Roy W. Menninger, Topeka, KS
Mary E. Mercer, Nyack, NY
Derek Miller, Chicago, IL
Richard D. Morrill, Boston, MA
Joseph D. Noshpitz, Washington, DC
Bernard L. Pacella, New York, NY
Herbert Pardes, New York, NY
Marvin E. Perkins, Salem, VA
David N. Ratnavale, Bethesda, MD
W. Donald Ross, Cincinnati, OH
Lester H. Rudy, Chicago, IL
David S. Sanders, Los Angeles, CA
Donald J. Scherl, Brooklyn, NY
Charles Shagrass, Philadelphia, PA
Miles F. Shore, Boston, MA
Albert J. Silverman, Chicago, IL
Benson R. Snyder, Cambridge, MA
David A. Soskis, Bala Cynwyd, PA
Jeanne Spurlock, Washington, DC
Brandt F. Steele, Denver, CO
Alan A. Stone, Cambridge, MA
Perry C. Talkington, Dallas, TX
Bryce Templeton, Philadelphia, PA
Prescott W. Thompson, Beaverton, OR
Joe P. Tupin, Sacramento, CA
John A. Turner, San Francisco, CA
Gene L. Usdin, New Orleans, LA
Warren T. Vaughan, Jr., Portola Valley, CA
Andrew S. Watson, Ann Arbor, MI
Joseph B. Wheelwright, Kentfield, CA
Robert L. Williams, Houston, TX
Paul Tyler Wilson, Bethesda, MD
Sherwyn M. Woods, Los Angeles, CA
Kent A. Zimmerman, Berkeley, CA
Israel Zwerling, Philadelphia, PA

LIFE MEMBERS
C. Knight Aldrich, Charlottesville, VA
Bernard Bandler, Cambridge, MA
Walter E. Barton, Hartland, VT
Viola W. Bernard, New York, NY
Murray Bowen, Chevy Chase, MD
Henry W. Brosin, Tucson, AZ
John Donnelly, Hartford, CT

Merrill T. Eaton, Omaha, NE
O. Spurgeon English, Narberth, PA
Stephen Fleck, New Haven, CT
Jerome Frank, Baltimore, MD
Robert S. Garber, Longboat Key, FL
Robert I. Gibson, Towson, MD
Paul E. Huston, Iowa City, IA
Margaret M. Lawrence, Pomona, NY
Harold I. Lief, Philadelphia, PA
Morris A. Lipton, Chapel Hill, NC
Judd Marmor, Los Angeles, CA
Karl A. Menninger, Topeka, KS
Herbert C. Modlin, Topeka, KS
John C. Nemiah, Hanover, NH
Mabel Ross, Sun City, AZ
Julius Schreiber, Washington, DC
Robert E. Switzer, Dunn Loring, VA
George Tarjan, Los Angeles, CA
Jack A. Wolford, Pittsburgh, PA
Henry H. Work, Bethesda, MD

BOARD OF DIRECTORS

OFFICERS

President
Jerry M. Lewis
Timberlawn Foundation
P.O. Box 270789
Dallas, TX 75227

President-Elect
Carolyn B. Robinowitz
Deputy Medical Director
American Psychiatric Association
1400 K Street, N.W.
Washington, DC 20005

Secretary
Allan Beigel
30 Camino Español
Tucson, AZ 85716

Treasurer
Charles B. Wilkinson
600 E. 22nd Street
Kansas City, MO 64108